Multimethod
Assessment of Chronic Pain

Pergamon Titles of Related Interest

PSYCHOLOGY PRACTITIONER GUIDEBOOKS

EDITORS
Arnold P. Goldstein, Syracuse University
Leonard Krasner, Stanford University & SUNY at Stony Brook
Sol L. Garfield, Washington University

Multimethod Assessment of Chronic Pain

PAUL KAROLY
MARK P. JENSEN
Arizona State University

PERGAMON PRESS

OXFORD · NEW YORK · BEIJING · FRANKFURT
SÃO PAULO · SYDNEY · TOKYO · TORONTO

U.S.A.	Pergamon Press, Maxwell House, Fairview Park, Elmsford, New York 10523, U.S.A.
U.K.	Pergamon Press, Headington Hill Hall, Oxford OX3 0BW, England
PEOPLE'S REPUBLIC OF CHINA	Pergamon Press, Room 4037, Qianmen Hotel, Beijing People's Republic of China
FEDERAL REPUBLIC OF GERMANY	Pergamon Press, Hammerweg 6, D-6242 Kronberg, Federal Republic of Germany
BRAZIL	Pergamon Editora, Rua Eça de Queiros, 346, CEP 04011, Paraiso, São Paulo, Brazil
AUSTRALIA	Pergamon Press, Australia, P.O. Box 544, Potts Point, N.S.W. 2011, Australia
JAPAN	Pergamon Press, 8th Floor, Matsuoka Central Building, 1-7-1 Nishishinjuku Shinjuku-ku, Tokyo 160, Japan
CANADA	Pergamon Press Canada, Suite No 271, 253 College Street, Toronto, Ontario, Canada M5T 1R5

Copyright © 1987 Pergamon Books Inc.

First edition 1987

Library of Congress Cataloging in Publication Data
Karoly, Paul.
Multimethod assessment of chronic pain.

(Psychology practitioner guidebooks)
Bibliography: p.
Includes indexes.
1. Intractable pain—Measurement. I. Jensen,
Mark P. II. Title. III. Series. [DNLM: 1. Pain.
2. Pain Measurement—methods. WL 704 K18m]
RB127.K29 1987   616'.0472   86-30634
ISBN 0-08-032377-4 (Hardcover)
ISBN 0-08-032376-6 (Flexicover)

British Library Cataloguing in Publication Data
Karoly, Paul
  Multimethod assessment of chronic pain.
  —(Psychology practitioner guidebooks).
  1. Intractable pain—Treatment
  2. Psychotherapy
  I. Title II. Jensen, Mark P. III. Series
  616'.0472   RB127

  ISBN 0-08-032377-4
  ISBN 0-08-032376-6 Pbk

Printed in Great Britain by Hazell Watson & Viney Limited, Member of the BPCC Group, Aylesbury, Bucks

This book is dedicated to friends

FRED KANFER

ERICA ROSS

PETER RUEHLMAN

MARTIN SLOANE

And more friends

MARK COLLINS

CYD GOODWIN

COREY MEADOR

NANCY NORTON

and JOAN PIASECKI

Contents

Preface and Acknowledgments

Strictly speaking, it is incorrect to assume that therapeutic interventions for chronic pain or any other clinical entity follow directly upon the knowledge of the current status of a disorder or syndrome. Rather, treatments are built on a reasoned understanding of the nature of the presenting complaint and its ramifications. Although in some disciplines it is possible to find 1000 qualified clinicians agreeing on a diagnosis, this does not mean that inference has been bypassed and that "reality" has been captured. It means only that the methods employed by that discipline for fixing belief are capable of yielding consensual understandings. As our colleague Gustav Levine has defined it, *science* consists of a set of procedures for minimizing the degree to which investigators are "free to kid themselves," and a reliable system for making and organizing basic observations is a formidable deterrent to self-deception.

Conversely, when experts differ in their appraisals of fundamental problems, when consensus is rarely achieved, and when reasoned understandings are free to vary, then we think it can be said that we are dealing with an enterprise not yet ready to label itself a science. In such a domain, problem solutions (e.g., therapeutic programs) are diverse and their effectiveness is typically controvertible. Anyone familiar with the evaluation and treatment of chronic pain must admit that current practices place that discipline squarely in the camp of the fallible, fledgling sciences. The intent of this guidebook is to provide an organizing framework and a compendium of methods for pain assessors — those whose observations provide the basis for the systematic treatment of chronic pain — in the hope that we might contribute, in some small measure, to the restriction of their freedom (to kid themselves).

While attempting to be up-to-date and comprehensive, we have omitted systematic explication of signal detection methods and of cognitive-behavioral procedures. We consider psychophysical pain scaling, through controlled nociceptive stimulation or magnitude estimation procedures, to be an important avenue for data generation and theory building; yet, it has not found widespread application in clinical settings. Cognitive and social psychological insights and procedures are likewise viewed as basic, if not essential, to any comprehensive pain assessment (see the Afterword), but they are as yet unsystematized and largely unstudied insofar as the psychometric properties of the various measurement methods are concerned. We trust that in the near future both of these approaches can be sufficiently evaluated in the clinical context to allow their widespread adoption by pain assessors.

Our task has been aided by many individuals, most of all our teachers—the clinicians and researchers whose work we have herein cited and the pain patients with whom we have both been privileged to work. Secondly, the atmosphere engendered by the faculty, students, and staff of the psychology department at Arizona State University has provided a most painless setting within which to work and grow. We are particularly indebted to Patricia Johnson, LaVaun Habegger, and Judy Sarrett, who diligently typed various versions of the manuscript.

Chapter 1
The Multiple Contexts of Chronic Pain

Chronic pain has been the subject of a good deal of general media discussion, research, clinical work, and policy decision-making, particularly in the last decade, during which time its economic, social, and personal impact has become especially salient (Bonica, 1981; Linton, Melin, & Götestam, 1984). Unfortunately, the subject has been studied largely in the manner of the proverbial blind men examining the elephant. The analysis of pain is multidisciplinary, but not interdisciplinary, in the sense that medical, psychological, and social perspectives are seldom genuinely integrated. Chronic pain remains, for many clinicians, a matter of temporally extended acute pain, with a pro forma recognition that, if a person hurts for a long time, there are inevitable emotional and vocational consequences. Even for those who acknowledge the multidimensionality of chronic pain, few guides are available for understanding how it differs qualitatively from pain in its more familiar, acute form. The purpose of this guidebook is to offer some preliminary conceptual markers as well as many practical suggestions for describing and quantifying chronic pain, building on the basic biophysical properties of nociception but extending beyond these in several necessary directions.

DIAGNOSIS-TREATMENT RELATIONSHIP IN CHRONIC PAIN

Chronic pain sufferers, like the chronically mentally ill, the intellectually retarded, or the physically handicapped, are seldom expected to "get better" or "function normally", in part because of the enormity of their encumbrances (presumed and actual) and partly as a result of the expense and marginal effectiveness of organized, professionally managed intervention programs. Clinically significant gains with such disorders, should they occur, are often bought at the expense of excluding as patients those individuals whose limited

1

personal and social resources mark them as highly likely to resist, or drop out of, treatment. In short, we seem unable to "win" with many such patient populations unless we "stack the deck" in our favor.

Treatment failures (or time-limited clinical successes) frequently spring from superficial patient data gathering and from the circumscribed (unidimensional) conceptual frameworks of the assessor/clinician. We tend, for example, to approach such patients in terms of either the distant past or the immediately perceived present, seldom seeking to understand the unfolding of their ideas, actions, and emotions over time or across settings. Piecemeal treatments, therefore, tend to follow from our scanty and disjointed assessments acting in concert with the economically motivated search for comparatively brief, low cost interventions.

In recent years, commentators have pointed to the critical, yet relatively neglected, link between pain assessment and pain treatment (e.g., Chapman, Casey, Dubner, Foley, Gracely, & Reading, 1985; Götestam & Linton, 1985; Karoly, 1985; Turk & Kerns, 1983) in an effort to introduce order and standardization into a field characterized by diversity and specialization. Following a biomedical model, most clinical practitioners have sought to systematize pain interventions around subtypes of pain patients identified by whatever physical and psychosocial factors reliably discriminate between them. Thus, for example, it has been suggested that pain sufferers differ in terms of whether and how much their pain is physiologic (acute or stress-related), pathogenic(disease or injury-based), and/or psychologic, the latter group representing the most intractable patients who can be further subdivided in accordance with a variety of categorizing schemes.

For example, Gildenberg and DeVaul (1985) array chronic "psychological" pain patients according to the extent of "sick role occupancy," varying from the assigned patients (acute pain patients whose physicians inadvertently locked them into the medical system), to the pure psychogenic pain patients, the overwhelmed patients (those whose inability to cope with life stress exacerbates their conditions), and finally to the need-to-suffer patients (patients with the worst premorbid histories, who offer the greatest resistance to change). Hendler, Viernstein, Gucer, and Long (1979) also employ four categories of pain patients: objective pain patients (those with a good premorbid psychosocial history and "organically definable lesions"), undetermined (those with a good history, but no identifiable pathology), exaggerated pain patients (those with a "minor" organic problem and a psychiatric difficulty), and affective pain patients (those with clear psychiatric difficulties and no known physiologic basis for their pain). Blumer and Heilbronn (1981), following and building on the observations of Engel (1959), who first described the pain-prone patient, sought to identify a "distinct psychopathologic condition" in patients with pain of "obscure origin." These authors, evaluating a series of 234 pain patients, asserted that they had indeed found a homogeneous group who are "basically needy, insecure, and guilt-ridden" and whose dependency needs are aroused by the onset of pain. Blumer and Heilbronn (1981) consider the pain prone disorder to be a "depression-spectrum disease" and recommended antidepressant medication in place of psychotherapy. Finally, the Emory University Pain Estimate Model (Brena, 1983), like the systems already described, examines the chronic pain patient from the key perspectives of pain duration, degree of demonstrable organic involvement, and psychological (personality and learning history) characteristics, in order to arrive at a "diagnosis" with presumptive implications for treatments, prevention, or both. The four classes of patients identified by the Emory model are illustrated in Figure 1.1, along with the scheme for assigning points for each scalable element.

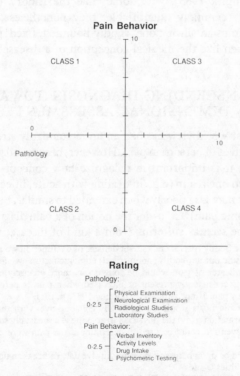

FIGURE 1.1. The Emory University Pain Estimate Model. Reprinted with permission from S. F. Brena "The medical diagnostic process". In S. F. Brena and S. L. Chapman (Eds.), *Management of Patients with Chronic Pain*, 1983. SP Medical.

Diagnostic systems such as those just mentioned have evolved to assist clinicians to: (a) predict the course and outcome of various pain and pain-related illnesses; (b) discriminate organic from psychogenic (functional) pain; and (c) match patients to appropriate therapeutic modalities. The success of these clinical endeavors has been spotty and inconsistent, with many studies suffering from methodological weakness (particularly the failure to establish the reliability of the diagnostic entities employed).

We believe, as do a number of critics of the pain measurement enterprise, that the benefits of categorical organizing schemes are outweighed by their disadvantages. To the extent that broad-based homogeneous subtypes of pain sufferers can indeed be discerned (acute versus chronic; good versus poor premorbid adjustment; the presence of clearly defined organic disease versus no known somatic elements), case management can certainly be tailored to the needs of the patient and to the skills of various specialists (surgeons, physiatrists, psychologists and psychiatrists, nurses, family counselors, and the like). Yet, despite the fact that categorical systems have a multidimensional appearance (consistent with the multiaxial spirit of the DSM-III; cf. Reich, Rosenblatt, & Tupin, 1983), with some (like the Emory University Pain Estimate Model) seemingly quantifiable, they nonetheless foster thinking about chronic pain as an all-or-none, rigidly bounded, fixed, person-centered phenomenon, much like the medical conception of a disease state.

TRANSCENDING DIAGNOSIS: TOWARD DIMENSIONAL ASSESSMENT

The biomedical world view has had an understandably strong and positive influence on the lives of persons in pain. However, because all world views have their limitations, it is important to recognize how concepts that have been proven effective in one realm (e.g., in dealing with acute, infectious diseases or pathologic states) may fare poorly when extended to similar, but nonequivalent phenomena (chronic pain). Consider the notion of a pain diagnosis. If a patient in pain were to be seen as suffering from a kind of disease, then:

- a search for the bodily (peripheral) site of damage or dysfunction would always be proper;
- an attempt to rule out nonbodily (nonmedical) etiologic factors would always be in order;
- a biological indicator of pain would be sought (or, more precisely, a "measurable body function that is consistently present or increased when pain is perceived and absent or decreased when pain is not perceived" (Brena, 1983, p. 101);
- the process of diagnosis would be minimally collaborative, with the patient essentially supplying information to aid the physician in arriving at a medically sound treatment plan;
- a placebo intervention could be used to determine if the pain were genuinely somatic or psychosomatic;
- the focus would be upon here-and-now descriptive data rather than upon the prediction of "future capabilities"; and
- the distinction between etiology and mechanism would be blurred (that is, factors that initiate the pain state would not be distinguished from those that influence the patient's ongoing interpretation of the meaning of his or her bodily experience; cf. Crue, 1983).

The present authors strongly believe that when an individual achieves the dubious status of chronic pain patient, it is the first duty of the assessment/intervention agent to seek to maintain that patient's integrity as a thinking, behaving, interacting, and growing (changing) human being who also happens to be feeling unpleasant bodily sensations (whether clearly or obliquely related to disordered medical states). Toward this purpose, we require a guiding conceptual model with the following attributes:

1. It should be *nonreductionistic*. If pain is objectified as a neurological event (measured as an evoked potential) or even a behavioral event (up time versus down time), then pain as a private experience (consciously felt, reported, and modified) is ruled out as a legitimate area of study. Similarly, if pain is reduced to a mental construction, the body and the environment lose their special meaning.

2. It should view chronic pain as existing along a continuum rather than characterizing it as a categorical variable. The influence of sensory events, emotions, thoughts, and actions can have an impact on the qualitative level and potential range of values along this continuum.

3. It should be multivariate, concerned with the configuration or structure of distinct elements that go to make up pain rather than focusing on isolated causes or effects.

4. It should seek to transcend linear causal logic in favor of a view of pain as emergent, as both a cause and an effect, and an organized complexity involving reciprocal relationships among biological, cognitive, and situational elements (cf. Elton, Stanley, and Burrows' 1983 circular model of pain).

5. It should not seek to represent the pain experience as context free, but rather as context dependent. By context, we do not simply refer to situations. Pain is also embedded in the contexts of the patient's goals, the clinician's expectations, the assessor's measurement model, and so on (see below).

6. The conceptual model should have direct treatment relevance by adopting a competency-based rather than solely a deficiency-based perspective on the patient. That is, the model should allow its users to address "what's right" with the patient as well as what is obviously dysfunctional.

7. It should provide for an active view, rather than a passive one of adaptation. The pain patient is seeking to make sense of, and accommodate to, his or her pain, and to make the pain experience congruent with his or her goals. Because chronic pain is such a debilitating condition, one whose body-centeredness fixes it squarely within the province of medicine, it is commonplace to find pain patients being treated, trained, educated, rehabilitated, and the like with minimal concern for self-determined learning and problem-solving.

8. The approach should emphasize process as well as content. What the pain feels like is critical: however so is how the sensory message is processed—not as an event that is simply fed into the system, but as an ever-changing product of the human capacity for representation, reflection, and self-guidance.

9. Knowledge, within the conceptual model, should be construed in relational rather than absolutistic terms. A pain threshold, a score on an MMPI subscale, and a request for analgesics are, by themselves, uninterpretable, decontextualized pieces of the pain puzzle, and like the pieces of any puzzle they are without value unless embedded in a recognizable network of relationships. And, finally . . .

10. The guiding conceptual approach should take into account that there is nothing to be gained by seeking to establish the final "objective" reality of felt pain. Rather it should recognize that chronic pain is a social construction just as much as it is a bodily reaction, and that it may profitably be seen as "the result of an active, cooperative enterprise of persons in relationship" (Gergen, 1985, p. 5).

The Pain Context Model (cf. Karoly, 1985) provides a base of understanding which we believe, meets the 10 criteria just noted for preserving the integrity of the individual suffering prolonged physical discomfort or pain.

INTERPRETIVE CONTEXTS OF CHRONIC PAIN

As professionals interested in understanding and assisting persons in pain, we share a common concern for justifying our beliefs and inferences about what it means when a patient says, "My pain is the worst it's been in 10 years, or "That medication I'm taking ain't worth a damn!", or "I feel I'm almost ready to go back to work." Although we may think about it less, we also need to justify our interpretations of X-rays, patient observation records, or pill counts, despite the seeming obviousness of these latter (so-called "objective" indicators. Whenever an actor sends a message to a receiver (a participant or audience), interpreters are faced with having to separate the sender's intent from the verbal and nonverbal message received. Why is this a problem? Sometimes an actor may not be fully aware of the intent of his message. Sometimes the listener is primed to accept only one of a number of possible alternative meanings. Sometimes the rules for interpreting the message are obscured by the vagaries of language or by the absence of sufficient background data on the kind of person the sender is, data that would allow the listener to be more certain of the correctness of his or her inferences. Pain patients, like other message senders, need to be interpreted in context.

That the role expectations of both the patient and caregiver can becloud the communicative context is illustrated by Meinhart and McCaffery (1983) in their excellent textbook on pain:

> Both the patient's and the nurse's beliefs about pain may preclude an accurate nursing diagnosis of the patient's pain problem. Thus, the patient ultimately may not receive adequate treatment for his pain. Some patients deny they have pain. Others cannot report their pain in an understandable way. Others will not report their pain. Still others may feel that the nurse knows their diagnosis and, therefore, whether or not they have pain, and that they would do something about it if they felt they could or if it were indicated (p. 12).

Similarly, Chapman and Wyckoff (1981) note the problem of word meaning as it is reflected in the pain complaint:

> Pain is almost always heard as a plea for help arising from a disturbed biological process, but it is often uttered to express moods and emotions or simply to evoke nurturance from others. In some cases, it can be used as an act of aggression to punish or blame others or even to accuse a therapist of failure ... Semantically, patients may use the word *pain* in any connotative or symbolic way that they choose, but physicians are expected to respond in terms of medical definitions and to provide only medical therapies (p. 34).

Is there a proper context for interpreting pain, one that will insure that caregivers (be they physicians, nurses, family members, or concerned friends) respond appropriately each from within his or her unique purview? A number of outstanding theorists working to disentangle the chronic pain problem have converged on the conviction that progress depends on the recognition that many factors, influencing each other reciprocally rather than unilaterally, contribute to the experience and expression of pain, and that no single discipline has all the answers (or even all the questions). Basically, the multidimensionality and complex causal structures inherent in modern conceptions of chronic pain (e.g., Chapman & Wyckoff, 1981; Melzack & Wall, 1965; Sternbach, 1968) are strongly tied to considerations of content, and direct themselves toward clarifying diverse pathways to pain perception and action. Improving our sense of where to look, however, does not necessarily enhance our understanding of why we are looking or what we should do with the data that have been gathered. As pain assessors we are coparticipants, not merely observers, and therefore, although there is no single best way to interpret pain, we can probably serve our patients better if we acknowledge that we are jointly engaged in creating the pain dimensions we seek to measure.

Does a surgeon create the herniated disk or the X-ray that reveals it? Of course not. But these are not equivalent to the low back pain that has been diagnosed and that takes on a life of its own in the minds of the physician and of the patient. Does the nurse create a patient's request for medication? No. However, as a participant in the very human drama of hospitalization, he or she becomes as much a part of what it means to be a pain patient as does the patient. Multiple contexts provide the background against which the sensory, evaluative, emotional, and behavioral aspects of noxious experience become figural, and help us to transcend the all-or-none, static, patient-centered conceptions of chronic pain that have therefore failed to enhance the quality of our patients' lives.

We consider four pain contexts, listed in Table 1.1, to be worthy of every assessor/clinician's attention. It should be understood that these are not presented as discrete, qualitatively unique agencies — such as body, mind, and environment — that are sometimes capable of cross talk. Rather, the contexts represent parallel or simultaneous levels of analysis, a four-dimensional systems world view with the potential to organize patient assessment and treatment.

Context I

The biomedical domain constitutes Context I. Although no more basic or real than any other perspective, the biomedical context is the most fundamental to our understanding of pain, in the sense that unusual bodily functioning is typically understood — within industrialized Western and Eastern societies — to be the rightful province of medicine. Although some forms of short-term, acute pain can be tolerated or self-treated and even considered nonpathologic (e.g., labor pain), prolonged pain, with its attendant suffering, is usually considered part of a patient's role, played out in a larger arena structured and controlled by the health professions. Biomedicine usually approaches pain assessment in ways analogous to the methods it uses to pinpoint other covert bodily events

Table 1.1. The Four Contexts of Chronic Pain

Context IV: *(Conceptual/Sociological Level)*
- Theoretical Approach
- Measurement Model
- Policy (Values) Orientation

Context III: *(Meaning/Relational Dimensions)*
- Temporal/Developmental
- Motivational/Rehabilitative
- Normative-Adjustmental (Mental Health)
- Environmental (Situational)
- Vocational (Task Specific)
- Familial
- Self-Perceptual/Self-Regulatory

Context II: (Focal/Experiential Dimensions)
- Sensory-Perceptual
- Affective (Emotion-Focused)
- Performance/Functional/Motoric (Behavioral)
- Interpersonal
- Verbal (Descriptive)
- Cognitive/Representational

Context I: (Biomedical)
- Medical and Surgical History (Present and Past)
- Physical Diagnosis Related to Pain Problems (e.g., Myofacial Pain, Peripheral Neuropathy, Causalgia, etc.)
- Medication Use (Present and Past Usage of Analgesics, Narcotics, and the like)
- Family Health History
- Biophysical/Neurochemical Status
- Doctor–Patient Relationships — Past and Present

(blood counts, CAT scans, electrencephalographic recordings, and the like). Although the medical system does not create pain signals within the body's interior, it nonetheless provides the most widely accepted, apparently scientific vocabulary in order to construct; the most widely accepted methods to treat; and the most likely arena in which to examine the unfolding of the chronic-pain lifestyle. Medicine concerns itself largely with the mechanics of pain, searching for the answer to the question, "Why does this patient hurt?," primarily at the organic level. Acknowledging that personality or perception may play a role in pain reactivity, medicine nonetheless assigns the task of understanding these components to psychiatrists or psychologists.

Consequently, as Scarry (1985) notes in her philosophical treatise on pain:

> physicians (often) do not trust (hence, hear) the human voice . . . they in effect perceive the voice of the patient as an "unreliable narrator" of bodily events, a voice which must be bypassed as quickly as possible so that they can get around and behind it to the physical events themselves . . . Thus, the reality of a patient's X-rayable cancer may be believed-in, but the accompanying pain disbelieved and pain medication underprescribed (pp. 6–7).

The objective of Context I is to "get around and behind", and also inside of, chronic pain. It is such an important and complex undertaking that we will devote Chapter 2 of this guidebook to its further explication.

Context II

If chronic pain is a medical construction, it is also a constellation of psychological attributes that serve to characterize the individual's experience of hurt and suffering and that also lend themselves to descriptive and quantitative analysis. Whereas Context I deals with where and why the person complains of pain, Context II focuses on what pain feels like, looks like, and signifies in the patient's life space. Whereas the Context I assessor may palpate a bodily area to determine the presence of myofacial trigger points, a Context II assessor (often, but not always, the same person as our hypothetical Context I assessor) may ask the patient to indicate the intensity of the experience of hurt by marking a line on a piece of paper, or may observe the sufferer as he or she engages in daily patterns of work, play, rest, or medication-taking activity — all to justify believing that a private, subjective experience has been at least partially understood. Referring to Context II as focal pain dimensions, the first author has described them as including:

> the immediate products of both the unpleasant sensation and what Beecher (1959) called the reactive component, as well as the extended processes that derive from the actions of the central nervous system (particularly the higher centers) and that produce the complex patterns of intrapsychic and social adaptation . . . (Karoly, 1985, p. 469).

Context II represents the heart of pain assessment for most researchers and nonmedical clinicians because it concerns itself with pain as it is experienced and expressed. (In discussing the idea of multiple interpretive contexts, we have encountered a tendency by some members of our audience to conclude that Context I refers to the physical or objective aspects of pain and Context II the mental or subjective side. We do not intend this sort of translation because we feel that such dichotomies are both clinically and conceptually unproductive. By establishing two discrete realms of reality [mind versus body and intangible versus tangible] we are forced to try to determine precisely how they occasionally interact. The relationship between what people do [or say], what they look or feel like, and what is verifiably true [action, appearance, and reality] is a philosophical rather than an empirical problem. Reality is neither in the body [and mind] of the pain patient nor on the physician's X-ray plate. Rather than choose sides in an unresolvable duality, we suggest that pain assessors consider the model articulated over a half century ago by philosopher Michael Oakeshott [1933], who argued: "experience is . . . a homogeneous whole within which distinctions and modifications may appear, but which know no absolute division" [p. 27]. Thus, the experience of pain [the subject of Context II] is the totality of pain from the patient's perspective, a reality that is both subjective and objective, underneath the skin and displayable, a process as well as a series of discrete outcomes.)

Key Assumptions of Context II: Pain as a Complex Perception

For most people, including scientists and researchers, pain is, more than anything else — an unpleasant sensory event whose most salient quality is its intensity (or its potential to arouse). Perhaps more attention has been paid to the assessment of the sensory intensity dimension than to any other single aspect of the pain experience (Melzack, 1983). It is not difficult to understand why the sensory signaling function of pain has so dominated theory, research, and practice — for the sensation of pain is both vividly real for the person who suffers it* and clearly analogous to other bodily systems, such as vision and hearing, whose mechanisms have increasingly yielded to empirical analysis dating back to the 16th and 17th centuries.

Over the years, clinicians and reasearchers have come to consider certain perceptual-sensory characteristics as central to the understanding of pain, including intensity; bodily location; onset; duration; spatial radiation; degree of associated hotness/coldness; type of pressure (sharp or dull); apparent depth; ease of detectability (threshold); the individual's general state of physiological arousal; the pattern of variation of these charcteristics; and the relationship of these perceptual experiences to environmental, cognitive, visceral, behavioral, and nervous system events (Meinhart & McCaffery, 1983; Melzack & Wall, 1965, 1983). The importance of each of these characteristics varies with the assessor's purpose, being particularly valued in formulating differential diagnosis and in assessing the effectiveness of specific pain treatments. (See Chapter 2.)

Pain is also an emotional experience, an affective response to a perceived stress that involves the cognitive, motor, and somatic systems (cf. Melzack & Wall, 1983). It is the potentially debilitating aspects of pain-related emotionality that assessors have traditionally sought to tap, (usually through questionnaires or, sometimes, observational recordings). An important conceptual advance in pain assessment is the recognition (by no means universal, however) that emotionality and its correlated approach/avoidance tendencies should be viewed as a fundamental dimension of pain rather than a psychiatric overlay.

---

*As Scarry (1985) so eloquently stated "for the person in pain, so incontestably and unnegotiably present is it that 'having pain' may come to be thought of as the most vibrant example of what it is to 'have certainty' . . ."(p. 4).

The third focal dimension, motor performance, is perhaps the easiest to quantify and is the subject of several well-researched observational recording procedures (to be discussed in Chapter 6). Because pain is part of a cognition-action system, making use of feedback and storage mechanisms, the inclusion of a behavioral dimension under the heading of pain as a complex perception is not at all out of place.

Similarly, our inclusion of an interpersonal or social component in Context II is consistent with a model (to be elaborated below) in which pain is part of an open system of interacting elements, one in which causes and effects are difficult to discern (and the idea of biopsychosocial explanations becomes central). Suffice it to say that pain as perceived and as enacted is subject to continued social and cultural influences.

The way in which patients verbally describe their pain experience also deserves to be established as a focal dimension worthy of study, if for no other reason than it is most often relied upon when assessing and conceptualizing the subjective aspects of pain. It is also important to note that modern psychological therapies for pain depend upon alteration of pain communication styles.

The final focal dimension, the cognitive-representational, has for too long been neglected in pain assessment. However, thanks to the gate-control model and the advent of cognitive-behavioral approaches to pain (e.g., Turk, Meichenbaum, & Genest, 1983), the importance of patients' appraisals, judgements, self-assessments, and modes of representing their "illness" and its effects is being recognized.

An exclusive focus on the physics of pain (that is, on its tissue-centered, psychosocially impenetrable nature) falls under the heading of nociception, which as Chapman and Wyckoff (1981) note, is "a neurological process of information transmission that is necessary for pain to occur, but not sufficient to explain pain as it is seen clinically"(p. 48). Philosophically, this assertion reflects the distinction between *peripheralist* versus *centralist* theories of pain (Crue, 1983; Meinhart & McCaffery, 1983), wherein one group (the peripheralists) sees the major or most salient aspect of pain as organic, with the psychological attributes being secondary (an overlay), and the other group (the centralists) sees the situation as reversed. The present authors are disinclined to the terms *peripheralist* and *centralist*, because they obscure the fact that investigators within both camps usually acknowledge the multidimensional nature of pain. Perhaps a better way of labeling the different stances is as linear versus systems centered. Both acknowledge sensory and psychological components in pain. However, the former assumes a "series of linearly chained processing steps," as Weimer (1977) calls them, wherein the sensation precedes and set the stage for whatever evaluational, motivational, or behavioral events might follow. Systems conceptions (e.g. those of Elton, Stanley, & Burrows, 1983; Engelbart & Vrancken, 1984; Melzack & Casey, 1986), however, view pain experience as psychologically penetrable, inherently involving a "dynamic interpenetration" of physiological, emotional, interpretative, linguistic, and social variables that cannot be reduced to any lowest common, physical denominator. The circular model of Elton, Stanley, and Burrows (1983) and the gate-control schematic of Melzack and Wall (1983) both illustrate the systems approach to the conceptualization of pain (particularly in its chronic forms) (Figures 1.2 and 1.3).

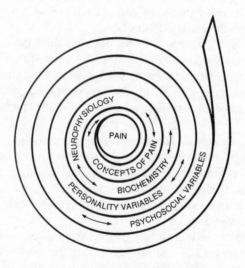

FIGURE 1.2. A circular model of pain viewed from above. Reprinted with permission from D. Elton, G. Stanley, & G. Burrows (1983). *Psychological Control of Pain*. Grune & Stratton, Inc.

Of all the extant conceptions of pain, the Melzack and Wall gate-control model is most responsible for illuminating the possibilities of Context II. Although the details will be considered in the next chapter, the schematic (Figure 1.3) clearly shows ascending (upwards from the periphery) and descending (downward from the central nervous system) influences, leading to the view that "the presence or absence of pain is determined by the balance between the sensory and central inputs . . . " (Melzack & Wall, 1965, p. 977). The projections from the brainstem reticular formation implicate the all-important role of arousal and attention in the total pain experience. The cerebral cortex and thalmus can also open or close the so-called pain gate. This

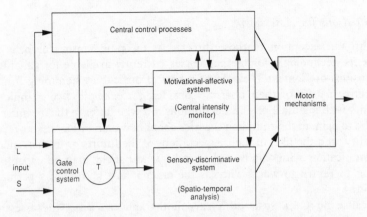

FIGURE 1.3. Conceptual model of the sensory, motivational, and central control determinants of pain. The output of the T cells of the gate-control system projects to the sensory-discriminative system (via neospinothalmic fibers) and the motivational-affective system (via the paramedial ascending system). The central control trigger is represented by a line running from the large fiber system to central control processes; these, in turn, project back to the gate-control system and to the sensory-discriminative and motivational-affective systems. All three systems interact with one another, and project to the motor system. From *The Challenge of Pain* by R. Melzack and P. D. Wall. Copyright 1982 by R. Melzack and P. D. Wall, Reprinted with permission of Basic Books, Inc. Publishers.

cortical involvement is of particular importance in understanding chronic pain because:

> . . . the individual's own unique thoughts, feelings, and memories can influence whether or not pain impulses reach the level of awareness . . . [Certain] memories are stored in the brain, and for the rest of his or her life, they are capable of influencing the transmission of potentially painful stimuli . . . Some types of chronic pain may be, at least in part, a "bad memory" (Meinhart & McCaffery, 1983, pp. 83–84).

Thanks to the work of Melzack, Wall, and their colleagues, there now seems to be ample neurologic (and not just experiential) evidence that pain consists not only of sensory but also of affective and cognitive components as well. Moreover, when pain is prolonged, whether there is evidence of tissue pathology or not, the system within which the pain exists widens to include social or interpersonal cues and consequences. That is, because pain may be displayed either motorically or verbally, it can be seen as a response capable of being strengthened or weakened by rewards or punishments, the attention or inattention emitted by significant persons in the patient's life (cf. Fordyce, 1976; Kremer, Sieber, & Atkinson, 1985; Sanders, 1979).

Implications for Assessment

With the exception of those directed at the pure sensory or behavioral elements, technologies or methodologies currently available for gauging the dimensions of Context II confront a host of difficulties stemming from the subjective nature of their quarry. Consider, for example, two chronic pain patients with identical physical conditions but who differ in the meaning they ascribe to pain, in their implicit theories about how pain influences work, play, sexuality, and the like, in their expectations of the future, or in their mode of communication with family and friends. One patient may be capable and willing to return to work, whereas the other is fast becoming a permanent invalid.

Because no CAT scan or X-ray photograph can assist the assessor in differentiating between such patients, other methods are needed. Much of this guidebook reviews and evaluates the procedures available, many relying on a self-report format, which elucidate the experiential or focal dimensions of Context II pain. To those who seek absolute objectivity in the measurement of pain, the widespread reliance on subjective data is sufficient to reject much of the contemporary practice of *algesimetry* (or pain measurement). It is the authors' contention that the acceptance or rejection of a chronic pain assessment procedure must not be based on any simple judgement about what constitutes good or bad science, but instead should follow from a consideration of why assessment data are needed and how they are to be used. These issues comprise what we call Context III.

Context III

Our third interpretive context is built around the guiding question: "What difference does the pain make?", and helps to clarify the varied uses to which pain status data can be put. An assessment program can hardly be considered finished after an understanding is obtained of either the pathophysiologic aspect of pain or its experiential character, because we have yet to determine what impact the pain has on the enterprise of living and growing. In short, we still need to determine what pain means, its relationship to important life tasks. In this vein, it has been said that true knowledge is knowledge of relationships; for our purposes, knowledge of pain implies an ability to relate measured pain to the varied processes of adaptation — to the patient's overall mental health, to the general quality of his or her life, and to specific, daily, goal-directed pursuits involving family, friends, work, play, self-improvement and spirituality, and contributions to the general welfare. In other words, chronic pain is a problem not just because it hurts, but also because the hurt or discomfort has important lifestyle implications.

Until recently, Context III has been largely implicit in pain assessment. A major contribution of the operant approach to pain management (e.g., Fordyce, 1976) has, in fact, been its clear demonstration of the situational embeddedness of pain complaints and behaviors. A person in pain also views the environment differently and, to the extent that he or she becomes self-absorbed or preoccupied, freedom of environmental movement becomes restricted and overall quality of life declines (cf. Diener, 1984).

Working in Context III, assessors can address the guiding question of "What difference does the pain make?" from at least seven distinct but related perspectives (Table 1.1). The fact that each of the six experiential aspects of pain (Context II), as well as the physical aspect, can impinge on each of the seven adaptational concerns of Context III means that there are actually no fewer than 49 ways of approaching this question. Fortunately, clinical pin assessors will rarely need to address all of the possible questions, although the present authors believe that many important avenues have, to date, been overlooked.

The Temporal/Developmental Dimension

As we have already noted, chronic pain does not emerge full-blown. Although many diverse factors may initiate pain sensations, it is generally believed that different patterns of adaptation to the pain, over the course of 6 months to 1 year after its onset, tend to set the patient on a path toward chronicity. What gives meaning to the pain experience is not simply its relationship to the passage of time, but rather to the internal and external events that occur over time. When, for example, early pain treatments fail to bring relief, patients may believe that their suffering is uncontrollable, leading to demoralization or a sense of helplessness. Similarly, the actions of significant others (family, friends, and physicians) may help to solidify a chronic pattern of pain complaints, inactivity, excessive medication taking, and the like, if the social environment provides attention, sympathy, financial compensation and other forms of "reward" contingent upon pain behavior (cf. Keefe & Brown, 1982; and Chapter 2 of the present volume for further details in the temporal aspects of chronicity). Therefore, it is important that the assessor seek to apprehend the pain problem with respect to not just its cause or its manner of expression, but also the unfolding of actions, reactions, beliefs, biases, and social transactions over time. Because continued surveillance of clients over long periods is typically not feasible, data on temporal patterns are usually obtained through interviews, recollections, and short-term diary keeping.

There is also a second sense in which temporal events become relevant to the interpretation of pain meaning; that is, the developmental changes in pain perception and expression occurring over the course of the life span. Although the state of the art of child pain assessment is less developed than adult-centered work (cf. Varni, Jay, Masek, & Thompson, 1986) and studies of the elderly tend to focus on anatomical and physiological deterioration, there is nonetheless a need to incorporate a developmental perspective when working at different segments of the age spectrum. The elderly become accustomed to physical pain and discomfort in their lives, and operate at reduced levels of activity. Underreporting of pain therefore becomes a problem for seniors, just as it does for young children who, by contrast, do not possess much knowledge about pain, its causes, or its treatments (cf. Ross & Ross, 1984).

The Motivational/Rehabilitative Dimension

In this chapter, we have argued that what an assessor learns about a patient depends on the mind-set or world view he or she brings to the task of understanding. When attempting to understand a complex system, such as a fellow human being in pain, we can adopt one of three stances first proposed by philosopher Daniel Dennett (1978) as a means of predicting the behavior of complex machines (also applicable to people). The design stance allows predictions to be based solely on "knowledge of or assumptions about the system's design" (p. 237), without needing to examine the actual processes that unfold within the system. We see instances of the design stance among psychologists when they prescribe standard "treatment packages" for pain patients, on the basis of group research showing that patients with problem X tend to respond favorably to treatment Y. The physical stance, which is more common in medicine (Context I), renders a prediction based on "the actual physical state of the particular object . . . worked out by applying whatever knowledge we have of the laws of nature" (Dennett, 1978, p. 4). Although both the design and the physical stances cover the mechanical aspects of a system's (person's) functioning, they do not do very well in the prediction of complex systems. Dennett's third stance, the intentional stance, captures the essence of what we mean by Context III's motivational level. As Dennett (1978) describes the intentional stance:

> One predicts behavior in such a case by ascribing to the system the *possession of certain information* and supposing it to be *directed by certain goals* and then working out the most reasonable or appropriate action on the basis of these ascriptions and suppositions (p. 6).

It is odd to think that some cognitive scientists and philosophers have been willing to assume intentionality on the part of machines (computers), but that clinicians have only recently (and often reluctantly) sought to examine the meaning of physical symptoms, such as pain, in the context of patients' goals and in their styles of processing goal-relevant information (cf. Leventhal & Nerenz, 1985).

For example, consider a patient with back and neck pain dating to a work-related injury who, for the last 2 years, has been in and out of the hospital and who claims to be unable to return to work because the "pain is so intense sometimes that I can't see straight!" The medical data are inconclusive, and programs of fluidotherapy, deep heating (shortwave diathermy), and massage have proven ineffective. The psychological profile reveals a man who reports intense pain, but who is not clinically depressed, does not limit his activities and, according to his spouse, is "no worse to live with than before the accident". The patient and his physician have agreed that surgery may be the only reasonable next step.

The descriptive accounts that emerge from the Context I and Context II assessments offer little direction for an intervention tailored to the needs of this particular patient. However, an intentional stance may provide the assessor with possibilities: Do psychometric instruments reveal a strong need or desire for control? Does the interview provide support for the view that the patient would rather collect his disability cheque than return to work? Was the patient unhappy on the job before the injury? (i.e. Is his overall quality of life thus perceived as improved even in the role of invalid?)

Among the most important intentional (or meaning) systems for a pain patient is that associated with his or her anticipated cure, recovery, or rehabilitation. A critical consideration for the patient involves his or her degree of involvement in the therapeutic regimen. Some patients want to be in the driver's seat, whereas others resent any professional who expects him to bear even part of the responsibility for dealing with the pain. Readiness or motivation to undergo therapy is often linked to the patient's general mental status, a topic represented in our third Context III dimension.

The Normative–Adjustmental Dimension

The dual hypothesis that pain leads to psychological maladjustment and that psychopathology is a precursor to chronic pain has a long history in clinical pain treatment and research. Much of the psychological and psychiatric assessment enterprise is directed at relating pain to mental health. As described in later chapters of this book, the usefulness of many traditional tests or assessment methods is equivocal when trying to establish a pain–mental health connection.

To date, however, numerous experiments have reported significant correlations between pain and various personality attributes, including self-esteem; depression; anxiety; locus of control; neuroticism; coping styles; extraversion; dependency; hysteria; and hypochondriasis (Elton, Stanley, & Burrows, 1983; Nigl, 1984). Because a psychological disturbance (as indexed by constructs such as those just noted) can result from or serve to predispose patients to, chronic pain patterns (and probably does *both* in many cases), assessors seeking to gauge the meaning of pain need be less concerned with chicken-and-egg questions than with obtaining an accurate picture of a patient's current state of mind and how it will impact on rehabilitative efforts.

The Environmental Dimension

Having discussed time as a critical interpretative dimension, we now turn to place. Our hypothesis is that the meaning of pain often varies as a function of where it is expressed or experienced. Two crucial settings for pain expression — the workplace and the home — will be discussed separately (in the next two subsections).

In general, however, the idea of interpreting pain in its place is limited mainly by our inability or unwillingness to obtain setting-specific information. The methods described in Chapter 6 for in situ assessment are far less prone to bias than are the retrospective data obtained through interviews or questionnaires. Unfortunately, they are also far more costly, and it is not surprising that "naturalistic" observations of nonverbal, motor "pain responses" have almost always been limited to hospital wards. The availability of automated, telemetric recording devices may help to naturalize the study of pain in real world settings, but it is unlikely that the average clinician will have the time and money to employ them. Assessment methods which may prove both cost-effective and accurate (but which remain largely untested) will be considered in Chapter 9.

The Vocational Dimension

To give the reader a sense of the different ways in which pain may be contextualized, we recommend that you think about the six experiential pain dimensions (Context II), listed in Table 1.1, and imagine first how they might be manifested in an office, a factory, or a retail store and, then, on a hospital ward. Consider what effect a verbal response such as "Boy, my back hurts" might have if uttered to a co-worker or employer as opposed to a ward nurse or physician. Consider the meaning of immobility (or functional incapacity) on a ward versus on the job. Try to imagine how an individual might cognitively reconstruct his or her pain problem based on recollections of 6 weeks on a pain unit versus 6 months on an assembly line.

Pain-mediated physical incapacitation and vocational disability are often related, but they are not synonymous. The same man whose disability prompts him to rely on his wife and children to do all the household chores — while catering to his every whim — may be motivated to perform his physically taxing factory job, for which his only relief is a beer or two or three with "the guys" after work. In addition, his self-reported pain intensity level and his sense of frustration might be the same in both settings, providing something of an enigma for the assessor whose predictions depend solely on the objective data. However as we shall discuss further in Chapter 8, apparent inconsistencies in the pain record can often be resolved by the adoption of the intentional stance toward the patient.

The Familial Dimension

Recently, the role of the family in the emergence and maintenance of the chronic pain lifestyle, as well as in its treatment, has come under increased scrutiny (cf. Block, Kremer, & Gaylor, 1980b; Rowat, 1985; Roy, 1985; Turk, Rudy, & Flor, 1985). As previously noted, the assessor needs to take developmental factors into account when in Context III, and the family is a major factor in providing youngsters with a relatively stable set of attitudes and habits of action, of language, and of thought regarding pain. Family dynamics are also influenced by the chronic pain of any of its members, often in the direction of disruption and restabilization around the sick members. We can, therefore, try the same thought experiment as before, only here imagining the six experiential pain dimensions played out in dyads such as husband–wife, father–son, mother–daughter. The family provides a unique relational framework within which to appreciate the changing meanings of chronic pain. Both assessment and treatment of pain in the family context are currently underdeveloped clinical arenas.

The Self-Perceptual/Self-Regulatory Dimension

Our discussion thus far has sought to show how the meaning of pain can be linked to its relationship to time, place, other persons, various life tasks or goals and the like, almost as if these relationships per se were a given fact of nature, and meaning flowed directly from them. Of course, implicit in all that we have stated is the assumption that the chronic pain sufferer is a symbol-manipulating organism, capable of (a) representing his or her beliefs, feelings, actions, and environments, and (b) reflecting on the way the information represented compares against various self-referential standards. The pain sufferer evaluates himself or herself socially, cognitively, physically, normatively, and morally, and seeks to either modify the standards or bring his or her actions, emotions, and beliefs in correspondence with socially acquired criteria of acceptability. Therefore, there is a self-perceptual and self-regulatory dimension along which to appreciate the relational meaning of pain. This is the all-important dimension that defines how the patient makes sense of pain (usually independent of the analysis of the physician).

Interestingly, assessors have both relied on and ignored patients' sense-making capacities over the years. That is, when patients complete attitude questionnaires or emotion checklists, when their motor responses are observed and tallied, and when they are asked to indicate their pain intensity, quality, location, and the like, we depend on their willingness and ability to make sense of their internal experiences, to transduce their physical sensations into *symbols* the rest of us can grasp, all the time taking the symbol manipulation at face value. Only recently have we begun to take pain-relevant cognitive activity (attributions, theory formulations, self-evaluations, plans, and the like) as a primary target of understanding and as a vehicle for intervention (cf. Turk, Holzman, & Kerns, 1986).

Context IV

The final interpretive context is perhaps the most abstract, referring not to the physical, experiential, or relational meanings of chronic pain, but to its ideological or conceptual embodiments. Context IV includes the perspective of the third party payer, the hospital administrator, and the state legislator, as well as the designer of the measurement tool used in pain assessment and the laboratory and applied pain researcher.

Although we do not have the space here to consider all of the cultural or social institutions with a vested interest in chronic pain, we can point out that over his "career" as a patient, the individual with prolonged pain may encounter not only physicians and nurses, but also psychologists, lawyers and the court system, insurance companies, clergy, nonprofessional support groups, and employee assistance personnel. Each specialty has a unique set of goals and values — their own "axes to grind" — regarding the patient's status.

Often implicit in the assessment or treatment enterprise is a theoretical stance. The physicalistic position of modern medicine is surely the best known viewpoint (described more fully in Chapter 2). Yet there are several extant models or conceptual frameworks, some only tacitly acknowledged, that influence how professionals make sense of chronic pain (and often how they expect their patients to do so).

A number of theoretical frameworks have been identified, many of which are compatible with each other. Among the models with psychosocial implications are: the communications model; the premorbid personality viewpoint; models built on the notion that pain provides legitimization for failure (cf. also self-handicapping theory); illness behavior theories; learning conceptions that distinguish between operant and respondent pain; models predicated on the interaction or transaction among multiple systems (cognition, behavior, physiology, and environment); and control theory (information-processing) conceptions. Once again, space limitations preclude a detailed summary of these varied conceptions of pain.(For more information, however, see Elton, Stanley, & Burrows, 1983; Main & Waddell, 1985; Meinhart & McCaffery,

1983; Melzack & Wall, 1983; Nigl, 1984; Slade, 1985; Turk, Meichenbaum, & Genest, 1983; Weisenberg, 1977.) The important point to be made here is simply that pain assessors should be able to make their theoretical assumptions clear and explicit, for if they fail to do so, they may make assertions incompatible with each other, with their own preconceptions, or with both.

The most detailed multiple systems view is that of Melzack and Wall (1983), the well-known gate control model (discussed further in Chapter 2 of this volume), which explains the characteristics of pathological pain syndromes and the role of central (psychological) mechanisms in pain perception. We believe that a compatible approach, based on cybernetic or information control theory, can describe the process dynamics linking the motives, skills, and actions typical of the chronic pain patient and to address the change mechanisms common to most psychologically based pain interventions (cf. Karoly, 1985; Turk, Holzman, & Kerns, 1986). For these reasons, we recommend the control theory approach as a general guide to conceptualization, and shall briefly outline one version as the final building block in our foundational account.

A CONTROL-SYSTEMS APPROACH TO CHRONIC PAIN

To achieve desired ends, humans actively engage their world — both the inner world of consciousness and the outer world of people and objects. Among the ends sought are optimal levels of somatic arousal, preferred self-evaluational states (ways of viewing oneself along such dimensions as competence, attractiveness, morality and the like), and environmental mastery (often in the service of the two previously noted goals). Thinking, feeling, and behavioral capacities represent the means available for the accomplishment of desired (or required) ends. Life goals are, in fact, rarely achieved; rather, the individual life course can be seen as consisting of cycles of goal-setting, goal achievement, disengagement, and resetting.

Although few would disagree with the foregoing general suppositions, the details can be presented in a host of distinct (and sometimes incompatible) ways. Until recently, investigators of chronic pain devoted comparatively little attention to the filling in of essential details in the relationship between pain and life goals as they are influenced by the cognitive, motivational, and behavioral capacities of pain patients. It has generally been assumed that chronic pain states or processes disrupt normal life pursuits, subjugating other goals to the goal of somatic-affective control (pain reduction or elimination) until, eventually, the patient's world is said to revolve around the pain despite his or her strongest wishes or preferences. Although broadly descriptive (as in the diagnostic formulations discussed in Chapter 2), such an account leaves out far too many connections to be very useful as a guide to assessment or clinical intervention. The present authors, who do not pretend to possess a complete model, will instead offer some brief statements of where we think the connections might be and of the factors that might serve to make and unmake them.

First, we shall assume that chronic pain patients, like the rest of us, are goal directed. To be goal directed requires both sensory and motor systems (the capacity to be aware of and act on the environment), as well as a representational system that reflects "the ability to create central representations of external events and to use them as a basis for behavior. . . ." (Oakley, 1985 p. 133). Unlike lower animals, which may also be presumed to represent the external world, humans possess the unique ability to represent themselves in relation to the outside world and in relation to the products of their own mind, depicting themselves in a "metaphorical space" that includes the past, the present, and the hoped-for or feared future. This capacity has been called self-reflective consciousness or the rerepresentational system (Oakley, 1985). Because of inherent limits to sensory intake and to motor output, it has been reasoned that the human brain evolved the rerepresentational system to serve as a sort of executive or supervisory means–ends coordinator, permitting complex action plans to be enacted, priorities to be set between competing goals, and emergencies (requiring immediate reactions) to be handled cost-effectively. Furthermore,

> It would appear that representations can be selected from the general pool of consciousness for re-representation within a system of priority processing. This system has a superior command over actions and is co-extensive with the realm of subjective experience (Oakley & Eames, 1985, p. 220).

By combining the current set of general concepts about consciousness with the previous discussion of Contexts II and III and the gate-control model, it should be possible to begin to reframe the notion of pain as a complex perception into one of pain as an information control/action system, the key elements of which are depicted in Figure 1.4.

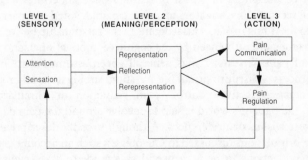

FIGURE 1.4.   A model of recurrent pain as an information control/action system.

To this structural model, highlighting the connections between sensation, meaning (subjective perceptual experience), and action, we need to add a set of hypothesized processes or control principles capable of explaining the clinical regularities characteristic of the chronic pain lifestyle, in a manner consistent with the 10 conceptual criteria outlined earlier in this chapter.

We may start with the basic assumption that the pain experience is

internally regulated in a closed-loop system organized so that the flow of *information* within it serves the purpose of keeping *momentary input* within the range of a preset (but not invariant) *standard* (Karoly, 1985 p. 484).

This assumption implies others. First, it elevates the concept of information to the level of a basic unit of analysis, in contrast to the physicalistic theories that emphasize the neural impulse or bioelectric force. Second, momentary input, which we will take to involve peripheral sensory stimulation of some sort, must be attended to before it is processed further. Attention serves to allocate energy for the task of continued processing or elaboration of informational sources. According to Leventhal and Everhart's (1979) parallel processing model, the individual preconsciously processes informational features of the pain stimulus (e.g., location, intensity, and quality,) at the same time as he or she processes emotional (distress-related) features. However, what determines which aspects of pain are processed further (paid attention to) so as to enter focal awareness? To answer this, we move to the third italicized term from the foregoing quotation, the notion of a reference standard (also referred to more broadly as a schema, prototype, or script). As Leventhal and Everhart (1979) have claimed:

Once an individual is no longer naive regarding pain, a noxious stimulus will retrieve and be integrated with the schematic memory of earlier pain experiences. To be very specific, we are arguing that the individual forms a schema, or categorical structure, that represents the informational and pain–emotion aspects of these experiences (p. 279).

The standard or schema is the key element of what we have labeled the meaning/perception level (Figure 1.4). It is, at its simplest, a goal or an image of a desired end state. Using the language of Figure 1.4, it is an abstract representation of perceived regularities in the external world and in the body, and of the relationship between the two (representation and rerepresentation, respectively). The pain patient, in the early stages of learning about and attempting to cope with discomfort, develops a theory or schematic model about his or her predicament, subject to the modifying effects of experience and continued thought (reflection). The model comes to serve as an organizing framework, guiding perceptions, expectancies, preferences, attentional foci, arousal, and action. We might say that when sensory inputs are processed at the schema level, the meaning is thus added. Furthermore, when a schema has been established and elaborated, it serves as a perceptual/attentional filter, partly determining what sensory events are allowed to reach consciousness. Therefore, if a person possesses a strong schema for the emotional components of pain, the continued experience of pain is possible even when no sensory message is available, as in the case of phantom limb pain (cf. Leventhal & Everhart, 1979; Melzack & Wall, 1983).

In addition to organizing perceptual selectively, memory, and arousal, the processes of representation, reflection, and rerepresentation eventually yield detailed scripts for the pain patient's behavioral and verbal exhibition of distress and for its inhibition. Dysfunctional (self-defeating) action structures for pain display and inhibition are as much a part of the chronic pain patient's clinical picture as are the emotionality, sensitivity to environmental stressors, personality changes, and related intrapsychic (internal) dysfunctions (feeling structures) that so often preoccupy assessors. The pain schema (or standard) can produce stability or change in action and thought through the control mechanisms of feedback and feedforward (i.e., by reinserting into the system the results of past performance and by proceeding with a planned action to a predetermined end point). In most chronic patients the feedback and feedforward mechanisms operate, but in the service of continued suffering and disability.

We might encompass many of the clinical features of chronic pain sufferers by asserting, from a control systems perspective, that (1) under the influence of reduced external stimulation and of sensory (organic) or schema-driven (acquired) processes, chronic patients tend to differentially monitor, encode, and interpret bodily activities as distressing (painful); (2) they tend to develop self-defeating cognitive-behavioral control strategies, including the denial of responsibility/capability for pain modulation, the pursuit of incompatible goals (e.g., to display and to suppress pain signals), and the schematic anticipation and avoidance of future suffering, leading to immobility-based muscular atrophy (and more pain); and (3) self-defeating patterns and conceptual models become strengthened through contingent social and financial rewards. Such a formulation is not antagonistic to any of the extant pain theories just described, nor does it disallow the fact that multimodal interventions for chronic pain have often seemed to work better than unitary treatments (i.e., biofeedback to correct faulty self-monitoring, relaxation for the conditioned arousal, self-efficacy to counteract negative expectations, and so on).

The present authors believe that the descriptive (organizational) power of the multiple context view, in concert with a control theory model of pain adjustment processes, can undergird an assessment enterprise that has, to date, proven extremely resistant to systemization. Readers are free to use the remainder of this guidebook as a simple catalogue of existing and promising measurement tools for chronic pain, fitting them into whatever conceptual schemes they may have already adopted.

CHAPTER SUMMARY

This introductory chapter aims to provide a clear set of assumptions about how to effectively and comprehensively think about chronic pain, with particular emphasis on alternate, equally valid but distinct levels of construing pain's multidimensional reality. Context II is the patient's reality, and the subject of most of the psychometric efforts undertaken in the last 50 years by both clinicians and laboratory researchers. Context III focuses on the meaning of pain as it is experienced and as this experience has impact upon adaptation. The Context III assessor seeks to relate the mechanics of pain and the varied ways in which pain is processed to its varied lifestyle implications. Finally, Context IV deals with the alternative theoretical realities around which professionals and administrators, researchers, and politicians tend to orient their thinking about chronic pain. A control-systems perspective was suggested as offering the greatest heuristic and organizational power as a model of chronic pain.

PLAN OF THE BOOK

To the superstructure presented in this chapter, the bricks and mortar will slowly be added in the chapters that follow. Chapter 2 highlights the physical aspects of pain perception and the unique perspective of modern medicine. It should make clear why the medical model is the place to start but not to end our assessment enterprise. Chapters 3, 4, 5, 6, and 7 provide a compendium of alternative methods for gauging the elements of Context II and the relationships of Context III. These chapters cover the essence of contemporary pain assessment methodologies, revealing their strengths and weaknesses. Chapter 8 is an effort to help the pain assessor integrate the diverse and often conflicting database that emerges from a comprehensive assessment program. Finally, in an afterword, we briefly discuss the problems confronting contemporary algesimetry and the prospects for the future.

Chapter 2
The Biomedical Context

Because most people make distinctions between the mind and the body, because pain is perceived as body-centered, and because clinical medicine is the chief discipline charged with bodily repair and restoration, it is not at all surprising (or inappropriate) that medicine has provided the archetypal interpretive context for pain. As noted in Chapter 1, medicine also teaches (socializes) us, both directly and indirectly, about the significance of pain and its modes of treatment. When adults take their pain to physicians (and other health professionals) and when children take their pain to parents (who have themselves been socialized by physicians), the medical contextualization process becomes relevant and figural. Although parents are the front line diagnosticians, for children, of "where and why it hurts", the assessment of these (and other) basic biophysical questions typically falls to experts in the evaluation and remediation of abnormal somatic conditions.

MEDICAL EVALUATION OF CHRONIC PAIN

As noted by Savitz (1985), the physician who seeks to understand a patient with major pain complaints

> should apply the usual model of history taking; physical examination; the ordering and assessing of appropriate lab, X-ray, and other ancillary tests; formulation of diagnoses; and formulation of treatment plan (p. 39).

Physicians require an organizing framework to both acquire and evaluate the utility of the data collected through interview, physical examination, and state-of-the-art laboratory testing. Knowledge of pathophysiology and its relation to mechanisms of sensory transmission and the use of pain classification schemes assist the physician in making sense of patients' pain problems.

26

The Acute–Chronic Distinction

Unquestionably, the most frequent differentiation between types of pain involves the labels *acute* and *chronic*. In many textbooks, the major distinguishing characteristic is time, that is, chronic pain is said to be pain that persists 6 months or longer. Although diagnosis based solely on temporal dimensions is useful, it is limited. As Crue, a physician and advocate of a time-centered assessment model, has noted:

> Most of us have been taught that the only difference between acute and chronic pain is the length of time it has persisted. We have thus often thought of chronic pain as a continuation of pain in the acute nociceptive input pain model. We have often unthinkingly confused etiology and mechanism . . . Physicians have long been aware that, as the pain continues over time, more and more central aspects, historically referred to as "functional overlay", inevitably become operative . . . (1985, p. xvii).

Practical, clinical experience as well as consideration of the gate-control and contextual models previously discussed, calls into question any one-dimensional approach to the acute-chronic differentiation. In fact, failure to clearly separate initial precipitating from current maintaining factors may also have ethical implications when, for example, physicians who fail to discover a clearcut biophysical source for the continuing complaint of pain essentially blame their patients, and discount their somatic experiences as purely psychological in nature (Gildenberg & DeVaul, 1985).

A fourfold characterization of acute versus chronic pain, based primarily on the work of Crue (1979, 1985), Pinsky (1978), Keefe and Brown (1982), Sternbach (1974), and others, is presented in Table 2.1. We believe that an initial classification based on pain duration, the presumed role of pathological bodily states, the manner in which the patient thinks about and reacts to the pain, and the treatment style and expectations of significant others represent a reasonable reinterpretation of the acute–chronic distinction, one that avoids the oversimplification often evident in the clinical literature. The foregoing account is not intended as explanatory or quantitative, but rather is a descriptive (qualitative) rendering, based on a great deal of accumulated clinical experience.

In the biomedical context, pain diagnosis is predicated on differentiating pain that is the result of either a psychiatric problem, a tissue-centered disorder (disease or injury), or the patient's history of lifestyle disruption secondary to intractable, persistent pain of unknown origin. Unfortunately, the science of pain assessment has not yet progressed to the point at which such clear differential diagnoses can reliably be made. However, some useful rules of thumb do exist. It is generally agreed, for example, that a chronic pain pattern does not occur full-blown, but rather develops (or evolves) as felt pain persists and as medical (surgical, drug-based, or other body-centered) interventions fail

Table 2.1.　Pain Classification Based on Duration of Complaint, Putative Causal Agent, Patient Coping Style, and Significant Other (Physician, Family) Reaction Patterns

---

Acute

Up to a few days' duration
Mild or severe
Cause(s) unknown or known
Presumed nociceptive stimulus
Sufferer expects relief based on medical interventions; extended coping efforts not seen as necessary
Physician expects pain complaints to decrease with healing of affected tissues (e.g., sunburn, toothache, and postsurgical pain)

Recurrent Acute (Intermittent)

Patient experiences variable pain-free intervals
Presumed nociceptive (tissue-derived) input from a pathological process (e.g., migraines, sickle cell crisis, arthritis, primary trigeminal neuralgia, and myofacial pain)
Physician expects continued therapeutic efforts to pay off

Ongoing Acute (Progressive)

Continued nociceptive input (e.g., from cancer)
Physicians willing to use potent narcotics
Patients often concerned about the effect of analgesics on chemotherapy
Treated like acute pain by patients and physicians

Prechronic

A few days' to a few months' duration
Similar to acute, except not viewed as an emergency
Known pathology
Physician concerned with use of narcotic medication (e.g., addiction)
Protracted healing process stressful (or, at least, autonomically arousing) to the sufferer
Patterns of coping originally elicited by internal events are coming under the control of situational variables
Some patients (with poor premorbid histories) are "at risk" to develop chronic intractable pain patterns

Chronic Benign (Persistent)

Nonneoplastic (noncancerous)
About 6 months in duration
No known pathology or nociceptive input
Patient is apparently coping adequately, has not made pain the center of his/her life
Physicians feel they can establish a working relationship with these patients

Chronic Intractable Benign Pain Syndrome (CIBPS)

Duration of 1 year and up
Physicians view patients as difficult to treat. Psychiatric referrals are common
Patients show physical decline (usually brought on by inactivity), psychological passivity (discouragement; depression), and excessive preoccupation with pain
Familial reward for "invalid" status (secondary gain) (For more details see text and Table 2.2)

Note. Table adopted from several sources (Crue, 1985; Keefe & Brown, 1982; Pinsky & Crue, 1984).

to provide relief. Therefore, the effective design and implementation of pain treatments, be they physical, psychological, social, or a combination of these, rests on the clinician's ability (a) to recognize clusters of patient characteristics and experiences that reflect dysfunctional learning and ineffective coping (chronicity potential or achieved chronicity), (b) to be a good medical diagnostician, and (c) to recognize his or her own role in strengthening or weakening the patient's style of pain adaptation.

Physicians working with pain patients rely on their ability to recognize the constellation of attributes constituting the chronic intractable benign pain syndrome (CIBPS), as outlined in Table 2.2, and on the knowledge of physical disorders commonly seen in the pain clinic, as outlined in Table 2.3 below. Psychiatrists and psychologists are also available for consultation, to help the physician gain an understanding of psychologicial problems as antecedents to or as consequences of particular pain syndromes.

Table 2.2.   Chronic Intractable Benign Pain Syndrome

A. *General Characteristics*

The chronic intractable benign pain syndrome (CIBPS) is defined as an ongoing problem with pain that:
  1. Cannot be shown to be causally related in the here and now with any active pathophysiologic or pathoanatomic process
  2. Has a history of generally ineffective medical and surgical intervention in the pain problem
  3. Has come to be accompanied by disturbed psychosocial functioning that includes the pain complaint and the epiphenomena that accompany it

B. *Epiphenomena*
  1. Substance use disorders of varying severity with their attendant central nervous system side effects
  2. Multiple operations or pharmacological treatments with their own morbid side effects separate from those related in (1)
  3. Escalating physical incapacity secondary to pain, anticipated pain, and fear that this increased pain is a signal of increasing bodily harm and damage
  4. Increasing hopelessness and helplessness as increasing dysphoria does not give way in the face of mounting numbers of "newer" or different therapies
  5. Conflicts with medical care delivery personnel (doctors, nurses, therapists, and technicians) with resulting dissatisfaction and/or different therapies
  6. Interpersonal conflict with significant others
  7. Unpleasant and lasting mood and affect changes
  8. Decrease in feelings of self-esteem, self-worth, and self-confidence
  9. Escalating psychosocial withdrawal and increased loss of gratification from these interactional inputs
  10. Decreased ability to obtain pleasure from the life process, contributing to profound demoralization and, at times, significant depression

Note. From "Intensive Group Psychotherapy." by J. J. Pinsky and B. L. Crue, 1984. In P. D. Wall and R. Melzack (Eds.), *Textbook of Pain.* Edinburgh: Churchill Livingstone (p. 823). Reprinted with permission, Longman Group, Ltd.

Table 2.3.   Disorders Seen in the Pain Clinic

Neurological Disorders
  Nerve lesions
    Posttraumatic neuritis
    Causalgia
    Postoperative neuromas
    Amputation stump pain
    Coccydynia
    Scar pain
    Nerve entrapments
  Postherpetic neuralgia (shingles)
  Trigeminal neuralgia (tic douloureaux)
  Sympathetic dystrophy
  Painful spastic states
  Thalamic pain

Musculoskeletal Disorders
  Low back pain (spondylitis, arthritis, failed disk surgery, etc.)
  Myofacial pain syndrome
  Paget's disease (with encroachment on nerves)

Ischemic Disorders
  Peripheral vascular disease (claudication)
  Angina pectoris

Neoplasm
  Direct invasion or compression of painful structures
  Metastases

Psychiatric Disorders
  Neurotic illness and mixed depressions
  Headache (some types)

Miscellaneous
  Dental pain
  Myofacial pain dysfunction syndrome
  Temporal mandibular joint arthritis
  Other facial pain
  Gout
  Chronic pancreatitis

Obscure
  Pain of unknown cause (e.g., obscure abdominal pain)

Note. Diagnosis of the Patient with Chronic Pain by H. Merskey, 1978, *Journal of Human Stress, 4,* 3–7. Reprinted with permission of the author, Harold Merskey, D. M.

Status of Contemporary Diagnostic-Classificatory schemes

Recent years have seen major advances in the way clinical pain is conceptualized. It is less fashionable for contemporary diagnosticians, who no longer view pain as a purely sensory event, to seek to disentangle psychogenic pain from true organic pain. Physicians who can discover no tangible signs of pathophysiologic involvement do not as readily dismiss pain patients as "crocks" or manipulators, as in past years. Table 2.1, outlining four types of acute and two styles of chronic pain, should clearly facilitate the process of treatment selection, referral to relevant professional resources, and posttreatment assessment. Indeed, on many occasions, the structure of the medical system is such that, by the time a patient is seen in a multidisciplinary pain center, the diagnosis of CIBPS is almost a foregone conclusion. Pathophysiology is minor or nonexistent. Severe psychopathology is ruled out. A history of long-term pain, multiple professional consultations, depression, anger, multiple unsuccessful operations and significant disruption of vocational, sexual, recreational, and interpersonal activities were all discovered by previous professional contacts.

Unfortunately, the process is rarely so cut and dried. First, the classification scheme presented in Table 2.1 is not exhaustive, nor are the categories mutually exclusive (two requirements for reliable classification). For example, it is not immediately obvious where patients with long histories of low back pain belong, or where to locate patients with diagnosable tissue disorders (such as arthritis or myofacial pain) who are currently receiving effective medical treatment but who are also experiencing some or all of the so-called epiphenomena associated with CIBPS (Table 2.2). Does "unknown origin" imply unknowable origin? Can we clearly distinguish when a patient is coping with pain or whether he or she is coping in ways that are maximally adaptive over the long run?

Diagnostic systems such as those discussed here and in Chapter 1 are best looked on as tentative, and their value is partly a function of their descriptive richness and partly the result of their prognostic (predictive) accuracy. Any system that mixes historical (pain duration), sensory (pain intensity or severity), psychological (coping adequacy), and physical (degree of tissue involvement) dimensions deriving from multiple data sources (self-report, observation, bioassay, and the like) is bound to be somewhat immoderate and overworked (cf. Karoly, 1985).

Furthermore, there is a substantial difference between talking about something and measuring it. Although both measurement and description share the common goal of communication, the unique aspect of the former is its focus on the use of numbers to provide quantitative analyses of objects or persons. Although careful metric or numeric analyses are involved in the laboratory tests used to determine the presence or absence of disease or pathology and in the quantification of patients' sensory experience of pain and discomfort, the schemes in Table 2.1 and in Figure 1.1 (the Emory University Pain Estimate Model) remain dependent on the diagnostician's qualitative, summary impressions (translating numbers into categorical judgments).

The fact that classification systems can be useful, even if built solely on the nonnumerical sorting of objects or events according to presumed discriminating features, is illustrated by the sheer predictive power of medical and psychological histories. Table 2.4 also illustrates how a cardiologist, carefully noting patients' verbal accounts of "where, when, and how chest pain hurts" and the relationships between painful sensations and other factors (such as physical activity, diet, and mood) can be aided in the important process of differential diagnosis.

Neurophysiology of Pain

Diagnoses, even when noncontroversial, do not give working physicians or biological scientists an answer to the fundamental questions of how and why pain hurts. The how and why of pain, as far as medical doctors are concerned, refer to its material, bedrock reality, its neurological and biochemical substrates. Although much progress has been made in classifying the mechanics of pain — some of the details of which will be outlined next — it is important that we again remind the reader that a comprehensive approach to chronic pain cannot rest on a reductionist base. (Paradoxically, then, one of Context I's greatest strengths is also one of its greatest limiting features.) However, to the degree that pain can be viewed as an event within the body, we can begin to understand it systematically through an appreciation of the larger bodily systems from which it emerges — the nervous (central and peripheral) and endocrine (hormonal) systems.

Early attempts to discover the inner workings of pain assumed a straight-through connection between the skin and cerebral "pain centers." From Descartes' 17th century conjectures to the 19th century physiologic studies of Muller and Von Frey, the notion of pain specificity carried the day (cf. Melzack & Wall, 1983, Chapter 9). Basically, it was argued that the skin contained pain-specific sensory receptors that carried information to specific brain locations through specific neural pathways. Free nerve endings were frequently suggested as the pain receptor sites. As Melzack and Wall (1983) point out, there were many relatively obvious problems with specificity theory (e.g., the degree of felt pain is often not proportionate to the amount of tissue injury, that pain often persists in the absence of sensory stimulation, or that damage to the brain centers that supposedly subserve pain experiences often fails to eliminate pain). The belief in the specificity viewpoint has nonetheless persisted until the present time because it, as well as the alternative peripheral pattern and central summation theories, reflected some fundamental physiologic realities (such as receptor specialization and neural coding of sensory events.) In addition, these theories were plausible to many researchers and clinicians, and they suggested various workable modalities of treatment. As we review next the contemporary anatomically, biochemically, and

Table 2.4. Pain Patterns Associated with Selected Cardiovascular Conditions

Condition or Disorder	Onset and Duration	Location and Radiation	Pain Quality and Intensity	Behavioral/ Psychological Signs
Pericarditis (inflammation of the pericardium)	Sudden onset; may last for days	Under the breast plate, left of midline; radiates to back	Mild ache to severe, knife-like, sharp pain	Pain decreases when patient sits up; pain gets worse with deep breaths, laughing, or movement
Angina (Latin word for sore throat; now refers to chest pain due to reduced blood flow, ischemia)	Gradual or sudden onset; lasts several minutes (up to one half hour)	Under breast plate; radiates to back, neck, jaws, arms, even to fingers	Mild to moderate "presssure"; sense of tightness or squeezing	Nausea, desire to void, belching, shortness of breath, apprehension; pain decreases when patient slows activity
Myocardial Infarction (reduced blood flow and cellular death in the coronary arteries; also called *Acute Heart Attack*	Sudden onset; lasts several hours	Under the breast plate; radiates to jaws, neck, back, shoulders, one or both arms	Persistent, severe pressure, deep sensation of crushing, squeezing or heaviness	Apprehension, feeling of impending "doom"; nausea, vomiting, fatigue, and/or shortness of breath; occurs even when person is not exerting himself

electrophysiologically informed concepts of pain transmission, it would be useful to bear in mind that the accepted wisdom of 1987, like that of 1887, is naturally constrained by the limitations of our methodologies, ethics, goals, and creative imagination.

Pain-Relevant Nerve Fibers

The term *nociception* refers to the process by which information about pain is carried from peripheral sense receptors in the skin and in the viscera to the cerebral cortex through networks of neuronal relays. Exteroceptors on the body surface and propioceptors within the body are specialized neurons that receive stimulation — mechanical (e.g., stimulated by pressure), chemical, electrical, or thermal (heat–cold sensitive). As Smukler (1985) notes:

> At their peripheral endings, these neurons are activated by inflammation, ischemia (obstruction of blood flow), and noxious mechanical, thermal, and chemical stimuli. However, these nociceptors may also be activated more proximally as they pass through sites of entrapment, the intervertebral foramena (apertures through the spinal canal), and the spinal canal. Finally, intrinsic disease of the nerve and root, that is, neuritis and radiculitis, may activate the nociceptors (p. 2; explanations added).

The body is equipped with mechanical nociceptors, heat and cold nociceptors at the periphery (so-called first-order neurons) which then connect with neurons in the spinal cord and medulla (second-order neurons) which carry the sensory message (in the form of an electrical impulse) to the thalamus, from whence third-order neurons carry the impulse to the cerebral cortex (cf. Martin, 1981). Nociceptors, therefore, have a specialized function, although they are not specific for the receipt of only pain signals.

Second-order neurons transmit their signals through two major upwards (ascending) systems: the dorsal column medial-lemniscal system and the anterolateral system. The former mediates position sense, touch, and pressure. However, the anterolateral system plays the major role in pain transmission (Figure 2.1).

At the bottom of the figure is a transverse cross-section of the spinal cord, notable by a region facing dorsally (towards the back, as opposed to the abdomen) that resembles horns. The anterolateral system originates in cells of the dorsal horns. In humans, there are two kinds of peripheral (first-order) fibers critical to pain perception, which enter the spinal cord dorsal horns from the various sense receptors. Shown in Figure 2.1 are A-delta and C fibers, the former being finely myelinated, the latter unmyelinated, but both small in diameter. A-delta fibers are distributed in the skin and mucous membranes of the body, whereas C fibers are responsible for about two-thirds of all sensory afferent messages (Kelly, 1981; Melzack & Wall, 1983). A second kind of fiber

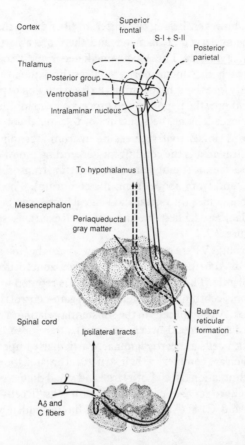

FIGURE 2.1. The anterolateral system of spinothalamic, spinoreticular, and spinotectal fibers, which convey information about pain to broad regions of the brain stem and diencephalon. Reprinted by permission of Elsevier Publishing Co., Inc., from D. D. Kelly (1981) Somatic sensory system IV: Central representations of pain and analgesia. In E. R. Kandel & J. H. Schwartz (Eds.), *Principles of Neural Science* (p. 210).

(not shown in the figure) is the relatively large diameter, myelinated A-beta variety. As far as pain perception is concerned, it is now believed that A-delta and C fibers tend to activate pain with the A-delta fiber producing fast, intense, localizable pain and the C fibers conducting slow, aching pain.

> When one bumps one's elbow, one feels a sharp pain immediately, the A-delta pain. Shortly thereafter, the individual experiences a dull, more aching C fiber pain. This latter type of aching or burning pain, which is considered more difficult to endure, is the type of pain that most patients with chronic pain syndromes experience (Meinhart & McCaffery, 1983, p. 37).

A-beta fibers, however, belong to a different fiber group than do the A-delta and C fibers, being larger in diameter and therefore able to conduct nerve impulses at a faster velocity. The A-beta–mediated, rapidly conducting afferent impulses that reach the dorsal horns as a result of touch or pressure (of a nonpainful variety) are thought to inhibit the transmission of pain messages. To better understand how the hypothesized process of pain inhibition operates, we need to take a closer look at the structure of the spinal cord.

The spinal cord dorsal root receives input from ascending sensory tracts, whereas the ventral area is the conduit for descending motor (action) tracts. It can be viewed as a feeling–doing relay center, getting transmissions from below (from the body) and from above (from the cerebrum). The butterfly-shaped structure, which includes the dorsal and ventral horns, can be usefully divided into layers or laminae (called the laminae of Rexed). A spinal segment is depicted in Figure 2.2.

Laminae I through VI are dorsal horn layers, with the first and second layers also identified by the formation of a definable zone called the substantia gelatinosa of Rolando. The substantia gelatinosa is reputed to play a key role in pain transmission, according to the well-known gate-control theory (Melzack & Wall, 1965, 1983). Although cells in the substantia gelatinosa project upward to the brain (through second-order neurons), they also connect to and communicate with cells in nearby laminae. Particularly important are the cells in lamina V, which are complex in their structural organization, responding to a wide range of stimulation (from both large and small diameter fibers). Lamina V cells are thought to serve as pain transmission cells (T cells). Small diameter fibers (A-delta and C) activate T cells, yielding a tendency for subsequent

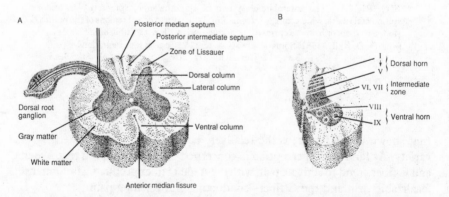

FIGURE 2.2.   A general organization of a spinal segment (A); a schematic view of the spinal gray matter (B). Reprinted by permission of Elsevier Publishing Co., Inc., from J. H. Martin (1981) Somatic sensory system II: Anatomical substrates for somatic sensation. In E. R. Kandel & J. H. Schwartz (Eds.), *Principles of Neural Science* (p. 173).

inputs to travel more readily to the brain. Large diameter fibers (such as A-beta fibers) also stimulate T cells, but a period of inhibition tends to follow activation. Thus, the basic idea of pain gating comes into being: the relative amount of activity in the small versus large diameter fibers influences the experiences of pain—small fiber activity facilitates, whereas large fiber activity tends to inhibit pain transmission. By analogy, small fiber activity opens the pain gate, whereas large fiber activity closes the pain gate (Melzack & Wall, 1965, 1983).

After passing the pain gates, nociceptive impulses travel over second-order neurons that ascend along the anterolateral tract (Figure 2.1). The major pain pathways in the anterolateral tract ascend to the thalamus, comprising the spinothalamic tract. This neuronal system has been called the pain tract because surgical sectioning of anterolateral fibers (an anterolateral cordotomy) produces relief from some painful conditions. In humans, the spinothalamic fibers cross before ascending to the thalamus. However, some fibers do ascend ipsilaterally, and transmission through these pathways may explain why pain returns to some patients who have had a cordotomy (Kelly, 1981). Another bundle of pain fibers in the anterolateral system is the spinoreticular tract, so named because its terminations are in a region of the brain stem called the reticular formation. Neurons in the reticular core are noted by the extensive network of connections they make, including the thalamus, hypothalamus, cerebellum, and cortex. Some pathways connect to the structures in the basal area of the brain called the limbic system, which is believed to mediate emotional responding. The midbrain periaqueductal gray matter shown in Figure 2.1 is another important structure insofar as pain modulation is concerned. Lesions in the area adjacent to the periaqueductal gray matter have caused animals to be hypersensitive to pain, whereas electrical stimulation of the lateral gray matter and nearby areas has yielded strong analgesic effects (Kelly, 1981; Melzack & Wall, 1983).

To complete our brief tour of the neurophysiology of pain, we must turn now to a consideration of central (cortical) control mechanisms. Sensory transmission, particularly pain gate activity, may be influenced by descending pathways originating in higher cortical centers. Psychological processes such as conditioning, attentional focus, expectancy, and emotionality (fear or depression) have been shown to influence the perception of response to pain. Melzack and Wall (1983) suggest that the dorsal column medial-lemniscal system heretofore ignored in favor of the anterolateral ascending system, could function so as to:

> activate selective brain processes such as memories of prior experience and pre-set response strategies that influence information which is still arriving over slowly conducting fibres or is being transmitted up more slowly conducting pathways (Melzack & Wall, 1983, p. 232).

As noted in Chapter 1, the gate-control model (Figure 1.3) provides physiologic justification for considering psychological determinants of the pain experience, especially in its incorporation of a motivational dimension and the central control trigger. These elements also have the virtue of permitting us to address medical oddities or pain states that would make little anatomical sense if all we had to work with was the old specificity model of pain transmission. For example, how would we account for injury without pain (as is often true of soldiers injured in battle), pain without injury, pain out of proportion to known damage, or pain persisting after healing or even after amputation of the damaged limb, if we did not have a model that offered a perspective on pain that allowed for multiple, interacting systems capable of integrating perceptual, motivational, and cognitive determinants of action? It is within such a model that psychogenic pain or CIBPS can be thoroughly investigated, as opposed to being dismissed as mere psychiatric overlay. Although physiologic and psychologic aspects of pain always co-exist, deciding on the relative importance of each is extremely difficult, as we shall see in the next section.

The Low Back Pain Patient: An Illustrative Case of Biomedical Assessment

John S. was a 37-year-old master carpenter, referred to a Comprehensive Pain Treatment Center by his family physician, who described him as having "low back pain secondary to muscle spasm which, having been self-treated and treated chiropractically each for 6 months, is now largely resistant to control via medication. Neurologic and discogenic findings are negative. The patient is mildly depressed and has not worked in a year".

Individuals such as John, with pain localized to the back (and sometimes to the head and/or neck) represent a significant medical and social problem. It is estimated that between 60 and 80% of the general population will at some time experience back pain of sufficient severity to interfere with their daily activities, and that 50% of all current disability-compensation payments are for persons with lumbar pain (Belkin, 1985; La Freniere, 1979; Nachemson, 1975, 1976). Low back pain costs the American wage earner 11 billion dollars annually, and is the leading cause of worker impairment (cf. Hoon, Feuerstein, & Papciak, 1985). In addition to its prevalence and cost, low back pain represents a genuine challenge to assessment. The referral of patients like John to a specialty pain clinic is today not unusual. Multidisciplinary centers are better prepared than are general practitioners to deal with both the medical and psychological difficulties that patients, sometimes called low back pain losers, tend to present.

Interview and Physical Examination

The neurosurgeon's interview and physical testing of John S. reveal many of the features of the chronic pain syndrome:

Diagnostician: You say you've had this pain for over a year now, and nothing much has
                       worked insofar as treatment is concerned. Does it hurt right now?
Patient (grimacing):   Oh, yes, doctor.
Doctor: Exactly what does the pain feel like?
Patient: Oh, do I have to talk about pain? It gets so damned tiring . . . well,
                       anyway, my back is just sore, more on the left side of my back . . . just sore
                       and tender.
Doctor: Is the pain steady, or does it vary?
Patient: It hurts a lot worse when I try to stand for a long time, or when I bend
                       over. I try not to do a lot of standing or bending.
Doctor: You lie down a lot.
Patient: Yes . . . yes, I have to, really.

After preparing the patient for the upcoming discomfort, the physician will
engage in a detailed physical examination and careful observational analysis.
The patient is led to an examination room while the physician notes unusual
postural characteristics (e.g., listing, unusual manner of walking, and sagging
abdomen). While the patient is disrobing, the physician checks for the presence
of pain equipment:

> This, in a back pain patient, may be a veritable cornucopia of paraphernalia including braces,
> corsets, orthotics for the shoes, lifts, canes, crutches, and transcutaneous stimulators (Belkin,
> 1985, p. 338).

Next, the patient is asked to walk, bend, raise and lower arms and legs while
lying down, stand on one leg, and perform other noninvasive tests designed to
inform the neurologist of specific sites of weakness or of possible neurological
involvement. Physical measurements of the lower extremities (e.g., calf and
thigh) may be taken to assess muscular atrophy. Deep tendon reflexes are also
tested. Tests for range of motion, both passive (patient is manually moved) and
active (patient is asked to initiate movements) are typically conducted, and
limitations noted. An extremely important component of the physical
examination involves palpation (i.e., the application of finger and palm pressure to parts of the patient's body), particularly on the spine, legs, and regions
of the back that are said to be the sources of pain. Palpation frequently reveals
trigger points or areas of extreme sensitivity that may have resulted from injury
to muscle or from visceral disease (Melzack & Wall, 1983). Pressure on trigger
points may reproduce the patient's presenting pain complaint or may cause
referred pain. Often an injection of local anesthetic into the trigger point can
completely alleviate the pain, suggesting muscle rather than nerve root
involvement (cf. Gildenberg & DeVaul, 1985).

Laboratory Tests

The neurologist's diagnosis depends on numerous laboratory tests, the
sophistication and reliability of which are remarkable. Blood tests, although not

usually indicated, can assist in differential diagnosis, if the pain is a result of anemia, infection, a tumor, or similar nonmechanical sources (Belkin, 1985). Most often used are various radiologic or radiographic techniques, including X-rays, radiculography (using radioactive media), computerized axial tomography (CAT) scans; NMR imaging; discography; and venography. Noninvasive, nonradioactive measures of assessment include electromyography (assessing muscle action potentials using electrodes); electronic thermography (a technique for measuring variations in heat emitted from the body's surface); and contact thermography (a nonelectronic system for producing thermograms) (cf. Belkin, 1985; LeRoy, Bruner, Christian, Filasky, & LeRoy, 1985).

Differential Diagnosis

From historical information, observation, physical examination, and laboratory test data, the medical diagnostician attempts to pinpoint the cause of the patient's pain and to render judgments relevant to the design of cost-effective treatment. It should be clear to the reader that back pain was selected as an example precisely because medical diagnostics alone often fail to yield clear-cut anatomical reasons for the patient's complaint, in as many as three-quarters of all cases. What the physician can do is to rule out causes that the data do not clearly support, a very important function indeed.

On the basis of up-to-date knowledge of the neurophysiology and musculature of the back and the spine, medical specialists seek to distinguish between a limited number of alternative causes of back pain. The spine may be the source of pain, if the vertebrae or intervertebral disk of the lower back are affected by fracture, dislocation, infection, inflammation, or metastic disease. Spine pain, or spondylogenic pain, arising from metabolic or malignant disease tends to be easier to diagnose than spondylogenic pain caused by mechanical derangement of spinal structures (Belkin, 1985). Pain may also originate in the spinal nerve root, particularly if it is compressed or irritated, in the synovial joints between the bony vertebrae, or in the spinal ligaments and paraspinal muscles. The last category, muscular/ligamentous pain, is important because the medical community tends (1) to diagnose it by exclusion, when laboratory tests fail to reveal structured abnormalities or the presence of disease, and (2) to attribute to it significant psychological overlay (cf. Dolce & Raczynski, 1985).

Back pain may also be the result of problems in areas other than the lumbosacral spine, including injury or disease of the abdomen and pelvis (so-called viscerogenic back pain) or vascular disease of the aorta or other arteries (vasculogenic back pain) (cf. Belkin, 1985).

Most back pain appears to be spondylogenic, with a large percentage of patients having muscular/ligamentous involvement. However, the assessment picture is complicated by the fact that many diagnosticians see a link between stress and muscular pain. Therefore, patients who have evidence of a herniated disk or nerve root compression may nonetheless experience prolonged muscle tension or reflexive spasms, as a result of stress due to incapacitation and inability to perform normal functions. This tension may lead to muscular/ligamentous involvement in addition to structural disorders already present. Similarly, ineffective coping may persist even after effective medical/surgical intervention has dealt with the precipitating disease or injury. The interaction of organic and psychological factors in back pain appears to be almost universal, precluding any clear-cut separation of physically based versus psychologically based pain. The future of chronic low back pain assessment, therefore, hinges on a recognition of the need to incorporate multiple descriptive and causal factors and to use assessment procedures capable of reliably indexing these factors (cf. Hoon, Feuerstein, & Papciak, 1985).

The remaining chapters in this guidebook will introduce a variety of methods that, taken together, offer the diagnostician a means of understanding pain not just as a symptomatic sensory reaction to tissue damage but also as a complex biopsychosocial phenomenon. These chapters should help us to appreciate why patients like John S. often differ dramatically in their experience of pain and their response to treatment, even when a definite tissue-centered agent, such as infection, injury, or tumor, has been medically confirmed (cf. Flor & Turk, 1984).

Chapter 3
Measures of the Subjective Pain Experience

The subjective sensations of pain, and the emotional responses that accompany these sensations, are what bring patients to clinicians. Clinical pain assessors depend on the patient's reports of subjective experience to develop both a diagnosis and a treatment plan, and on reports of changes in pain sensations to gauge treatment effectiveness. To assess the experiential dimension of pain (Context II), several self-rating scales and questionnaires have been developed. The immediate pain experience tapped by these scales can be roughly divided into four categories: how much it hurts (magnitude or intensity); how the individual responds emotionally to the pain experience (affective quality); what the pain feels like somatically (sensory quality); and where it hurts (location and spatial distribution).

MEASURES OF SUBJECTIVE PAIN INTENSITY

The most common measures of subjective pain intensity include the Verbal Rating Scale, the Visual Analogue Scale, and the Numerical Rating Scale. Less common measures include the Behavior Rating Scale, the Picture Scale, the Tourniquet Pain Test, and various other cross-modality matching methods.

Verbal Rating Scales

A Verbal Rating Scale (VRS) is a list of adjectives that describe different levels of pain intensity such as *mild* and *moderate*. The pain patient is asked to consider the list and choose the adjective that best describes her or his pain. The number of levels of intensity represented in these scales varies widely from as few as 4 to as many as 15. Table 3.1 provides examples of several different verbal rating scales.

Table 3.1.   Verbal Rating Scale Pain-Intensity Measures

Four-Point Scale (from Seymour, 1982)	*Four-Point Scale* (from Joyce, Zutshi, Hrubes, & Mason, 1975)
• No pain • Mild • Moderate • Severe	• No pain at all • Some pain • Considerable pain • Pain that could not be more severe

Five-Point Scale
(from Frank, Moll, & Hort,
  1982)
• None
• Mild
• Moderate
• Severe
• Very severe
	Five-Point Scale
	(from Kremer, Atkinson, &
	  Ignelzi, 1981)
	• No pain
	• Mild
	• Moderate
	• Horrible
	• Excruciating

Twelve-Point Scale
(from Tursky, Jamner, &
  Friedman, 1982)
• Not noticeable
• Just noticeable
• Very weak
• Weak
• Mild
• Moderate
• Strong
• Intense
• Very strong
• Severe
• Very intense
• Excruciating
	Fifteen-Point Scale
	(from Gracely, McGrath, &
	  Dubner, 1978a)
	• Extremely weak
	• Very weak
	• Weak
	• Very mild
	• Mild
	• Very moderate
	• Slightly moderate
	• Moderate
	• Barely strong
	• Slightly intense
	• Strong
	• Intense
	• Very strong
	• Very intense
	• Extremely intense

The usual method of scoring VRSs is to rank the words in order of intensity level, and then give the lowest-intensity adjective a score of 1, the next a score of 2, and so on until each word has a number associated with it. The number that corresponds to the adjective chosen by the patient represents his or her pain intensity score.

An alternative method of scoring VRSs using a cross-modality matching (CMM) approach is designed to provide a numerical estimate of pain that more closely approximates the patient's current perception, by anchoring the pain judgments to familiar physical modalities (Gracely, McGrath, & Dubner, 1978a; Tursky, Jamner, & Friedman, 1982). This scoring procedure involves asking patients to indicate the severity of pain that each word represents, with severity being equated to any one of several modalities, such as the loudness of a tone or the length of a line. The ratings for each word (or an average of the ratings if more than one is used) serve as the VRS scores. The major advantage of this scoring system is that, unlike the ranking method, it does not assume an equal interval between the intensity levels indicated by the successive words on the scale.

There are two major drawbacks to the cross-modality matching method. First, because patients must rate every word of the VRS before the scale can be used, patients may find it tedious to comply with the measurement task (Ahles, Ruckdeschel, & Blanchard, 1984). One way of increasing compliance is to forego the cross-modality match, and simply assign standardized scores that represent the average for each word given by groups of individuals (cf. Gracely, McGrath, & Dubner, 1978a; Tursky, Jamner, & Friedman, 1982; Urban, Keefe, & France, 1984 for lists of scores for specific words). Unfortunately, most lists were produced by non-patients in response to experimental pain, and there is evidence that chronic pain patients may rate the intensity of pain words differently than do acute (i.e., postoperative) pain patients (Wallenstein, Heidrich, Kaiko, & Houde, 1980). In the one available set of average scores developed from chronic pain patients, the scores developed from chronic pain patients differed up to 10 percent from one another, suggesting that the scores obtained from CMM methods may be less precise than originally thought (Urban, Keefe, & France, 1984).

In addition, scores produced by the CMM and ranking methods may correlate so highly that they contain essentially the same information, thereby making the use of the more complex and time-consuming CMM method unnecessary for estimating pain intensity (Hall, 1981). Therefore, we suggest that clinicians use the simple rank scoring method for the VRS. This method should provide clinicians with the information they are really after, whether or not their patients' pain is increasing, decreasing, or staying the same following treatment.

Verbal rating scales have several strengths. They can be extremely easy to administer and score. Ease of comprehension renders compliance rates for these scales as good or better than that for other intensity measures under most conditions. A final strength is that they have consistently demonstrated their validity as measures of pain intensity by: (a) yielding positive and significant correlations with other measures of pain intensity (Ahles, Ruckdeschel, & Blanchard, 1984; Downie, Leatham, Rhind, Wright, Branco, & Anderson, 1978; Jensen, Karoly, & Braver, 1986; Kremer, Atkinson, & Ignelzi, 1981; Ohnhaus & Adler, 1975; Woodforde & Merskey, 1972), (b) yielding relatively low correlations with measures of other pain constructs (Andrasik, Blanchard, Ahles, Pallmeyer, & Barron, 1981), and (c) demonstrating sensitivity to treatment effects (Fox & Melzack, 1976; Ohnhaus & Adler, 1975; Rybstein–Blinchik, 1979).

A common criticism of verbal rating scales is that they are less sensitive than the visual analogue scales to be described, because they do not provide sufficient response categories to permit the assessment of small changes in pain intensity. The VRS with only four response categories clearly does not allow for the variety of pain intensity experienced by pain patients. However, in measuring pain intensity in groups of patients, research performed to date indicates that under different conditions, neither the visual analogue scale nor the VRS is consistently more sensitive to treatment effects (cf. Joyce, Zutshi, Hrubes, & Mason, 1975; Ohnhaus & Adler, 1975).

Visual Analogue Scales and Graphic Rating Scales

The Visual Analogue Scale (VAS) consists of a straight line, usually 10 cm long, whose ends are defined as the extreme limits of pain. For example, one end may be defined as no pain, whereas the other may be defined as pain as bad as it could be. A VAS that has descriptive points between the extremes labeled with words or numbers, such as mild or severe, is called a Graphic Rating Scale (GRS). To quantify their pain, patients are asked to make a mark across the 10-cm line at the point that best indicates perceived severity. To score both scales, the distance from the no-pain end to the mark provided by the patient is measured. This distance defines the patient's pain intensity score (Figure 3.1).

A strength of the VAS is that it has demonstrated validity as a measure of pain intensity, by virtue of: (a) its positive relation to other measures of the intensity construct (Downie et al., 1978; Elton, Burrows, & Stanley, 1979; Jensen, Karoly, & Braver, 1986; Kremer, Atkinson, & Ignelzi, 1981; Ohnhaus & Adler, 1975; Seymour, 1982; Woodforde & Merskey, 1972); (b) lesser correlations to measures of other subjective components of pain (Ahles, Ruckdeschel, & Blanchard, 1984); and (c) sensitivity to treatment effects (Joyce, Zutshi, Hrubes, & Mason, 1975; Seymour, 1982; Turner, 1982).

The VAS displays three problems as a measure of pain intensity, however. First, measurement of pain intensity using a VAS requires two steps: (a) the estimation of the pain by the patient in terms of distance on a line, and (b) the careful measurement of the mark made by the pain patient. The second step not

Visual Analogue Scale

No pain _____ Pain as bad as it could be

Graphic Rating Scale

No pain _____ Pain as bad as it could be
     Mild   Moderate   Severe

FIGURE 3.1 Visual analogue and graphic rating scale measures of pain intensity.

only creates an extra possible source of error, but also requires extra time on the part of the assessor. A second problem is that users need to be careful not to employ photocopied versions of the scale, because photocopying usually changes the length of the line, making comparisons between the original and photocopied versions more difficult. Finally, older patients appear to have difficulty using visual analogue scales (Jensen, Karoly, & Braver, 1986; Kremer, Atkinson, & Ignelzi, 1981). Because of these problems and the existence of other valid measures of pain intensity, we suggest that the VAS not be employed as a primary measure of pain intensity in adult clinical populations. Conversely, the VAS is one of the few effective methods for use with young children (cf. Varni, Jay, Masek, & Thompson, 1986).

Numerical Rating Scales

A third common method of pain intensity assessment, called the Numerical Rating Scale (NRS), involves asking pain patients to rate their pain from 0 to 10 or 0 to 100, with the zero representing no pain and the 10 or 100 representing pain as bad as it could be. Whatever number the patient states, represents the pain intensity measure for that patient.

Numerical rating scales have consistently demonstrated their validity as pain intensity measures by their positive and significant correlation with other measures of pain intensity (Downie et al., 1978; Jensen, Karoly, & Braver, 1986; Kremer Atkinson, & Ignelzi, 1981; Seymour, 1982; Wallenstein, Heidrich, Kaiko, & Houde, 1980), and their sensitivity to treatment effects (Chesney & Shelton, 1976; Kaplan, Metzger, & Jablecki, 1983; Seymour, 1982; Stenn, Mothersill, & Brooke, 1979). Numerical rating scales are easier to understand and use than VASs, so they can be used with a great variety of patients. They are also extremely easy to administer and score. These advantages indicate strong support for the use of numerical rating scales. Of the two (11-point versus 101-point NRS), the 101-point NRS probably should be chosen, because it provides more response categories.

Other Intensity Measures

Pain intensity measures that have been used by researchers but which have yet to find widespread use among clinicians include the Behavior Rating Scale, the Picture Scale, the Tourniquet Pain Test, and other pain estimation procedures.

Behavior Rating Scale

The Behavior Rating Scale (BRS) was first developed by Budzynski, Stoyva, Adler, and Mullaney (1973) as a measure of head pain. An adaptation of this scale

Table 3.2. Behavioral Rating Scale of Pain Intensity

Behavioral Rating Scale
- No pain
- Low level pain that enters awareness only when I pay attention to it
- Pain exists, but can be ignored at times
- Pain exists, but I can continue performing all the tasks I normally would
- Very severe pain that makes concentration difficult, but allows me to perform tasks of an undemanding nature
- Intense, incapacitating pain

Note. Adapted from Budzynski, Stoyva, Adler, & Mullaney (1973). EMG biofeedback and tension headache: A controlled outcome study. *Psychosomatic Medicine, 35,* pp. 484–496.

is illustrated in Table 3.2. We call this instrument the Behavior Rating Scale because it asks patients to rate the intensity of their pain in terms of its effects on their behavior.

The BRS has demonstrated its validity as a measure of pain intensity through its significant correlation with other measures of pain intensity and its lesser correlations with measures of other subjective components of pain (Andrasik, Blanchard, Ahles, Pallmeyer, & Barron, 1981; Jensen, Karoly, & Braver, 1986), as well as by its demonstrated sensitivity to treatment effects (Budzynski, Stoyva, Adler, & Mullaney, 1973).

The BRS may also be more meaningful to some patients because it provides behavioral markers with which to judge pain (Collins & Thompson, 1979). However, because the BRS assesses pain intensity in terms of its effects and not how it feels, it is best to consider the BRS an indirect measure of intensity. This conclusion is consistent with the finding that the BRS shows the weakest relation to a composite measure of pain, when compared with other intensity measures (Jensen, Karoly, & Braver, 1986). In addition, the BRS provides relatively few response categories.

Picture Scale

An additional scale developed to assess pain intensity was described by Frank, Moll, and Hort (1982). The scale, called the Picture Scale (PS), employs eight line drawings which illustrate facial expressions of persons experiencing different levels of pain. To measure pain intensity, the eight pictures are presented to the patient in a random order, and the patient is asked to choose the picture that best illustrates his or her pain experience. Scoring the PS is simple. Each picture is associated with a number from 0 to 7, depending on the degree of pain intensity illustrated. The number associated with the picture chosen by the patient represents his or her pain intensity score.

One strength of the PS is that its use does not require that the patient be verbally fluent. Therefore, it has the potential to be useful as a measure of pediatric pain. However, although the PS has demonstrated some degree of validity, both through its significant relationship to a VAS and a 5-point VRS (Frank, Moll, & Hort, 1982), as well as through sensitivity to treatment effects (Mann, Kimber, Diggins, Jenkins, Vandenberg, & Currie 1984), the scale has yet to gain wide acceptance by clinicians, and it is not yet clear how it may relate to other measures of pain. The expressions illustrated on the PS appear to be very affect-laden, so the scale may be closely associated with the affective component of pain. Additional research with the PS is therefore indicated before it can be highly recommended as a measure of pain intensity.

Tourniquet Pain Test

The Tourniquet Pain Test (TPT) involves inducing ischemic pain in the arm of the pain patient. A pressure cuff is applied to the upper arm of the patient and inflated. The patient is then asked to operate a hand exerciser at a fixed rate. The procedure is accompanied by a slowly increasing deep pain ". . . similar to that of many pathological pains" (Sternbach, 1983, p. 27). The patient is asked to continue to operate the hand exerciser and indicate when the induced ischemic pain matches his or her clinical pain level. The patient is then asked to continue until pain tolerance is reached. This procedure produces three pain measures: (a) clinical pain level (the elapsed time in seconds for the patient to indicate that the ischemic pain matches the clinical pain); (b) pain tolerance (the time it takes the patient to indicate that he or she has reached the limit of tolerance); and (c) tourniquet pain ratio (the clinical pain level divided by the pain tolerance and then multiplied by 100). The first of these measures is the one presumed to be most associated with subjective pain intensity.

One advantage of the TPT over other matching tasks is that the stimulus to which patients attempt to match their clinical pain intensity is experimentally produced pain measured over time, rather than a physical modality that is merely an analogue, such as the length of a line.

Unfortunately, problems with the TPT limit widespread use among clinicians. These problems include: (a) The TPT may not be sensitive to treatment effects (Sternbach, Deems, Timmermans, & Huey, 1977); (b) Variables that may be difficult to control, such as the effort patients put into the hand exercise, influence the pain-intensity measure (Moore, Duncan, Scott, Gregg, & Ghia, 1979); (c) The method is time-consuming relative to other pain-intensity measures; and (d) The presence of an observer is required to monitor patient activity throughout its duration. In addition, the procedure involves inducing pain in a person who may already be suffering a great deal. Therefore, unless the clinician has some clear reason to use the TPT, and until future research supports its superior reliability and validity over those of other measures, the TPT probably should not be considered the measure of choice in the assessment of pain intensity.

Other Cross-Modality Matching Measures

For the clinician who requires intensity measures other than those already discussed, alternative methods are available. These include asking pain patients to match their intensity level to the frequency of a sound (Peck, 1967; Woodforde & Merskey, 1972), the length of a light bar (Adriaensen, Gybels, Handwerker, & Van Hees, 1984), and the loudness of a tone (Adams, Brechner, & Brechner, 1979). Although the scores obtained using these methods generally show a significant relationship to other measures of pain intensity and tend to be sensitive to treatment effects also measured by other measures, their drawbacks include the need for someone other than the patient to be present for the measure to be made and the need for some form of audio or visual equipment.

A recent comparison of several pain-intensity measures indicates that most of the scales just described (including the NRS-101, VRS-4, VRS-5, VAS, and BRS-6) all provide adequate measures of the intensity construct (Jensen, Karoly, & Braver, 1986). Because all are psychometrically adequate, the criteria for selecting one scale over another involve primarily practical issues such as the ease of administration and scoring, sensitivity (as defined by the number of response categories provided), and relative ease of subject comprehension of the scale. On the basis of these criteria, we prefer the NRS-101 because it is extremely easy to administer and score, it provides enough response categories (101) to be adequately sensitive to changes in pain level, and older patients do not appear to have greater difficulty with the measure. Another scale we recommend is the 6-point BRS, which can provide a unique and important assessment of pain intensity as it relates to the perceived behavioral effects of pain.

MEASURES OF THE AFFECTIVE COMPONENT OF PAIN

The importance of the affective dimension of pain has been emphasized in most recent conceptualizations of pain and pain assessment (cf. Melzack & Wall, 1983).

Two of the most common methods for measuring the suffering caused by pain are Verbal Rating Scales and the affective subscale of the McGill Pain Questionnaire. The latter instrument will be discussed in the next section. Two VRSs that have been developed for measuring the suffering caused by pain are illustrated in Table 3.3. They consist of adjectives describing increasing amounts of discomfort and suffering. Like those for pain intensity, these verbal scales may be scored in three ways: (a) the ranking method, which involves giving each word a score associated with its position in the list; (b) the cross-modality matching (CMM) method, which involves asking patients to indicate the

Table 3.3.   Verbal Rating Scale Measures of the Affective Component of Pain

Twelve-Point Scale (from Tursky, Jamner, & Friedman, 1982)	Fifteen-Point Scale (from Gracely, McGrath, & Dubner, 1978a)
● Not unpleasant	● Bearable
● Bearable	● Distracting
● Tolerable	● Unpleasant
● Uncomfortable	● Uncomfortable
● Distracting	● Distressing
● Unpleasant	● Oppressive
● Distressing	● Miserable
● Miserable	● Awful
● Awful	● Frightful
● Unbearable	● Dreadful
● Intolerable	● Horrible
● Agonizing	● Agonizing
	● Unbearable
	● Intolerable
	● Excruciating

degree of unpleasantness on a numerical or linear scale, and using the number stated, the length of the line drawn, or an average of the two as the score associated with each word (cf. Tursky, Jamner, & Friedman, 1982); and (c) the standardized score method, which incorporates the average ratings of the words on the VRSs by individuals experiencing laboratory (i.e., nonclinical) pain.

No study has directly examined the relative merits of scoring affective VRSs using the three scoring methods outlined. Given the compliance problems already noted with the CMM method when using VRSs to measure pain intensity and the potential difficulties associated with published average scores, we recommend the simpler ranking method until the superiority of another method is adequately demonstrated.

Some preliminary evidence exists for the validity of verbal rating scales as measures of the affective component of pain. Research generally indicates that verbal scales of suffering (a) correlate more with measures of other affect-laden constructs than with measures of pain intensity, and (b) are more responsive than measures of intensity to treatments designed to reduce the affective response to pain (Ahles, Ruckdeschel, & Blanchard, 1984; Andrasik, Blanchard, Ahles, Pallmeyer, & Barron, 1981; Gracely, McGrath, & Dubner, 1978a and 1978b).

SELF-RATINGS OF THE QUALITATIVE ASPECTS OF PAIN

The McGill Pain Questionnaire

The McGill Pain Questionnaire (MPQ; Melzack, 1975) is designed to provide information on three hypothesized dimensions of pain: the sensory (e.g., temporal, spatial, pressure, and thermal aspects), the affective (e.g., tension and fear aspects), and the evaluative (e.g., overall severity of the pain experience). The MPQ consists of a list of 78 adjectives, divided into 20 subclasses. Each subclass contains two to six words and is intended to reflect a specific quality of the pain experience. Sixteen of the subclasses comprise the items for the three dimensions of pain, with the sensory dimension represented by 10 subclasses, the affective dimension represented by 5 subclasses, and the evaluative dimension represented by 1 subclass. The remaining 4 subclasses consist of unclassified words, thus creating a "miscellaneous" subscale of pain. Patients are asked to choose no more than one word from each subclass that best describes their pain. If no word in a particular subclass describes the pain, the patient may omit the response. Each word in the 20 subclasses is associated with a specific score, ranging from 1 to 5, based on the average degree of pain intensity assigned by groups of physicians, patients, and students (Melzack & Torgerson, 1971).

According to Melzack (1975), the MPQ must be carefully administered to be reliable. Careful administration consists of reading the instructions to the patient and observing the patient as he or she fills out the questionnaire to insure that (a) no more than one word is selected per subclass, and (b) the patient understands that a word from every subclass does not have to be chosen. Also, because some of the words in the MPQ may be difficult for some patients to understand, someone needs to be present to define words when necessary. The MPQ requires 15 to 20 minutes to complete by patients who have not taken it before and 5 to 10 minutes by those experienced with it.

The MPQ yields several different scale scores. First are the pain-rating indexes (PRI(S)) calculated by summing the scale values of each word chosen. Scale values are the average rating of the word, as rated by groups of students, physicians, and pain patients (Melzack & Torgerson, 1971). A PRI(S) may be calculated either within a dimension of pain, thus creating a PRI(S)-affective score, a PRI(S)-sensory score, and the like, or across all dimensions, creating the PRI(S)-total score. Similar scores may be calculated by summing the rank values of the words chosen. These scores are designated PRI(R) and also may be calculated either within a dimension or across all the dimensions of pain. A third score, the number of words chosen (NWC), is calculated by simply summing the number of subclasses the patient uses to describe his or her pain.

Perhaps the greatest strength of the MPQ is that for the first time it allowed the quantification of many separate components of the subjective pain experiences. The value of measuring these multiple components has been demonstrated in a number of experiments. First, the MPQ was shown to reflect organic aspects of pain (Agnew & Merskey, 1976; Leavitt & Garron, 1979a). Second, the PRI-affective scale score has been shown to be useful in differentiating patients who demonstrate psychiatric disturbance from those who do not (Kremer & Atkinson, 1981; Kremer, Atkinson, & Kremer, 1983). The MPQ has also been successful in discriminating among patients who have different kinds of pain. Using the questionnaire, Dubuisson and Melzack (1976) were able to correctly classify 77% of patients suffering pain from cancer, degenerative joint disease, menstruation, a phantom limb, arthritis, a tooth, and posthepatic neuralgia. Finally, the MPQ has demonstrated validity as a measure of pain through the sensitivity of its subscales to treatment effects (e.g., Melzack & Perry, 1975; Rybstein-Blinchik, 1979).

Unfortunately, current evidence is not sufficient to allow adequate evaluation of the reliability of the MPQ. Although research suggests patients may tend to choose similar words to describe their pain over time (cf. Graham, Bond, Gerkovich, & Cook, 1980; Melzack, 1975), estimates of the stability and internal consistency of the subscales of the MPQ have not been provided.

A more serious concern with the MPQ involves the lack of evidence for the validity of the sensory and evaluative subscales of the measure. For example, factor analyses of the MPQ indicate that the scale measures from four to six dimensions in different pain populations (cf. Burckhardt, 1984; Byrne et al., 1982; Crockett, Prkachin, & Craig, 1977; McCreary, Turner, & Dawson, 1981; Prieto et al., 1980; Reading, 1979). In addition, a recent confirmatory factor analysis of the MPQ indicates that the three subscales are closely associated with one another and may not be measuring distinct aspects of pain (Turk, Rudy, & Salovey, 1985). These findings had been predicted to some degree by Melzack (1975) when he first introduced the MPQ and stated directly that, "The pain questionnaire so far is, to be sure, only a rough instrument" (p. 294).

Variations of the McGill Pain Questionnaire

At Melzack's (1975) suggestion, researchers have attempted to refine the MPQ so as to enhance its utility and validity. Such refinements have varied from altering how the questionnaire is administered and scored, to developing new questionnaires based to a large degree on the original MPQ.

One drawback to the MPQ as it is now scored is that comparisons between the three subscales are difficult. Using the ranking method of scoring, for example, the maximum PRI(R)-sensory score is 42, whereas the maximum PRI(R)-affective score is only 14. To make the scores more comparable, some researchers divide each subscale score by the maximum possible for that score (i.e., PRI(R)-sensory by 42, PRI(R)-affective by 14, and PRI(R)-evaluative by 5), producing subscale scores that always vary between 0 and 1. This scoring system has an advantage over the traditional system in that it makes subscale scores directly comparable without altering the amount of information provided by the subscale scores.

In a more complex system, Charter and Nehemkis (1983) altered both the administration and the scoring of the MPQ. Their first change was to place each subclass of words in the MPQ along a series of 10-cm visual analogue scales, with one per subclass. The word representing the lowest rank is at one end, and the word representing the highest rank is at the other end of each VAS. The other words of each subclass are placed between the two extremes at a distance proportional to their average intensity score, as initially measured by Melzack and Torgerson (1971).

Charter and Nehemkis (1983) describe several scale scores that may be calculated from the VASs. First is the Average Pain Intensity (ATP) which is computed by summing the scores for each subclass within a pain dimension and dividing this sum by the number of subclasses in that dimension. Since Charter and Nehemkis (1983) have incorporated the four miscellaneous subclasses of the MPQ into the sensory and affective dimensions, the divisors are 13 for the sensory dimension, 6 for the affective dimension, and still 1 for the evaluative dimension. The ATP is closely related to Melzack's (1975) PRI. A second score has no analogous measure in the traditional scoring of the MPQ. It is called the Average Pain Intensity–Word Classes Chosen (APC) and is calculated by summing the scores from the VASs and dividing this sum by the number of word classes chosen, rather than by the total number of word classes within each dimension. Unless a patient chooses every word class, the ATP score for a particular pain dimension will always be less than the word class APC score. (*Note*: Because there is only one subclass for the evaluative dimension, ATP–evaluative [ATP–E] will always equal APC–evaluative [APC–E].) A third measure is the percentage of words chosen (PWC). The PWC computed for the sensory and affective dimensions are called PWC-S and PWC-A, respectively, and the PWC computed for the total scale is called PWC-T. The PWC-T is analogous to the NWC of the MPQ scored in the traditional way. Charter and Nehemkis (1983) recommend that the PWC not be calculated from the evaluative dimension because it is made up of only one word group. Finally, the APT minus APC differences score can be calculated as an alternative measure of the number of subclasses chosen by the patient. In fact, as Charter and Nehemkis (1983) have pointed out, correlations between the APT–APC difference and PWC scale scores are very high (0.92 or higher) for the sensory and affective categories.

There are several advantages to the scoring method proposed by Charter and Nehemkis. First of all, like the other alternative scoring methods already discussed (e.g., dividing the PRI subscale scores by the total possible PRI subscale scores to make PRI[R]-E, PRI[R]-S, and PRI[R]-A comparable), it allows for a more direct comparison of sensory and affective subscores. Second, the APC measure allows an alternative, and perhaps more valid measure of the severity of sensory and affective perceptions. By assessing the average severity of subclasses for only those subclasses that are chosen, a more precise measure of the severity of experienced perceptions is obtained.

Charter and Nehemkis (1983) note that the scores calculated using their system may be obtained without the use of visual analogues and they have provided a way of converting traditional MPQ measures to their scores. If the Charter and Nehemkis (1983) scale scores are desired, the assessor must choose between the VAS procedure and converted traditional MPQ measures. Unfortunately, there has not been sufficient research to support the validity of one method over another.

The major weakness of the Charter and Nehemkis (1983) scoring method is that it does not address some of the problems associated with the traditional MPQ, such as the need for assessor presence to explain the scale and define words, the difficulty of some of the words, and the lack of sufficient evidence for the validity and reliability of the MPQ. Therefore, although the alternative scoring methods provide some improvement on the utility of the subscale scores obtained from the MPQ, they do not necessarily provide more valid measures of the constructs the MPQ is designed to measure.

Other Scales Based on the McGill Pain Questionnaire

To alleviate some problems associated with the MPQ, several pain scales, each based to a large degree on the MPQ, have been developed. The first was a card sort by Reading and Newton (1978). Beginning with the original list of pain descriptors examined by Melzack and Torgerson (1971), Reading and Newton (1978) narrowed the list down to those descriptors used most often by a group of women with pelvic pain. Sets of three descriptors were selected to represent 10 specific subclasses of pain, and these 10 sets were organized into four dimensions: sensory, affective, temporal, and evaluative. Cards with two words per card were then made, and the patient is asked to sort the cards depending on which of the words (top or bottom) best describes the pain.

A factor analysis revealed that the card-sort procedure measures three factors, two of which are made up primarily of the subscales created a priori (evaluative and sensory subscales), indicating that these two subscales may be internally consistent and relatively distinct from each other (at least for the population of subjects in the study, that is, women with pelvic pain). The scale thus shows promise as an alternative to the MPQ. However, future research with the scale is necessary to demonstrate the degree of its reliability and validity in other pain populations.

Hunter (1983) developed a scale specifically for headache patients. She reduced the original list of descriptors on the MPQ to a list of frequently used words (27) and added three words not on the MPQ but used frequently by headache patients. The 30 descriptors in the Headache Scale are presented to the patient so that each can be rated with regard to the degree that it describes a patients's pain on a 4-point Likert scale. The Headache Scale was given to 100 headache patients, and seven subscales were derived empirically through cluster analysis.

A discriminant function analysis showed that the 30-item Headache Scale could correctly classify 74% of migraine and tension headache sufferers, indicating a fair degree of discriminative validity. Like the card-sort technique developed by Reading and Newton (1978), the Headache Scale shows potential as a measure of the subjective qualities of pain. However, because it is new, much of the evidence required to judge its psychometric properties is lacking. Specifically, reliability estimates for the subscales, cross-validation of the cluster analysis, and evidence for validity of the individual subscales are all necessary before the Headache Scale may be adequately judged.

Finally, a Low Back Pain Questionnaire was developed by Leavitt, Garron, Whisler, and Sheinkop (1978). This scale consists of 74 words from the MPQ that were endorsed as descriptive of pain at least 6% or more of the time in a group of back pain patients. The respondent is asked to examine each word, and indicate whether it describes his or her pain. The words on the questionnaire are divided into seven subscales based on factor analysis of the responses provided by the initial group of 131 back pain patients. One of the subscales consists primarily of affective words, a second is a combination of mild affective and sensory words, and the rest all describe various sensory dimensions of the pain experience.

The instrument contains several improvements over the original MPQ. Because each word is judged by the pain patient, the number of items on the subscales increases, and scales with more items are generally more reliable than scales with fewer items, providing each item makes an independent contribution to measuring the construct of interest. However, reliability data (either test-retest stability or internal consistency) are not yet available. In addition, although one study showed validity for the low back pain questionnaire as a general measure of pain by demonstrating that some of the scales were sensitive to treatment effects (Leavitt, Garron, Whisler, & D'Angelo, 1980), basic research examining the specific meanings of each is still lacking.

There is a clear need for a valid and reliable measure of the qualitative aspects of the pain experience. Currently, several promising scales may be used to assess these aspects. However there is a paucity of evidence for the reliability and validity of most of these measures. Of the scales that are currently available, we recommend continued use of the MPQ, despite its problems, which hopefully will be resolved with more research. Because the MPQ has a longer history, its properties and drawbacks are more well known than are those of other scales that are currently being developed.

ASSESSING PAIN LOCATION: THE PAIN DRAWING

The pain drawing provides an excellent way of assessing where the patient experiences pain. The test stimulus is simple: a line drawing of the front and back views of the human body. After being shown the stimulus, patients are asked to indicate the location of their pain on the line drawings. Instructions vary regarding how the patient is to indicate the pain. For example, Melzack (1975) asked patients to indicate the location of external (i.e., surface) pain by writing the letter E on the drawing and to indicate internal (i.e., deep somatic) pain with the letter I. Ransford, Cairns, and Mooney (1976) asked pain patients to indicate four qualities of pain or discomfort on their drawings using the following symbols: — for numbness; *oo* for pins and needles; *xx* for burning; and // for stabbing pain. Others (e.g., Toomey, Gover, & Jones, 1983) ask their patients to shade in the areas of the body that are "in pain".

Toomey, Gover, and Jones (1983) divided their line drawing of the human body (as well as line drawings of the face and jaw because they assessed many facial pain patients) into 32 regions. They found that the number of regions shaded was related to many important pain-related constructs, including various scores on the MPQ (NWC, MPQ-sensory, and MPQ-total); self-report of time spent reclining; interference of pain with basic activities such as walking, working, socializing, and recreation; the number of health care professionals consulted; and medication use. The number of sites in pain was not related to pain intensity or chronicity. These results suggest that the total area of the body in pain is an important variable to consider in addition to the intensity of pain. In a subsequent study, these same investigators found that the site of pain (head and neck, low back, both head and neck and low back, and neither) was related to the interference of pain with daily activities, that is having low back pain or low back plus head and neck pain was associated with greater activity interference (Toomey, Gover, & Jones, 1984).

Using a rating system similar to that of Toomey, Gover, and Jones (1983) Margolis, Tait, and Krause (1986) divided the pain drawing into 45 regions. Patients are asked to shade in any area that is in pain. Using a plastic template, the pain drawing is scored by summing all of the areas that include at least some shading. In addition to this raw score, Margolis et al. (1986) calculated a weighted pain drawing score by summing the percentage of body area represented by each region that has some shading in it. Clerical staff with minimal training were able to score the pain drawings with a high degree of reliability. However, because the two scores obtained from the pain drawing were closely related ($r = 0.97$), indicating that they both carry the same information, we recommend that the simpler raw (i.e., unweighted) score be used as a measure of body area in pain.

A second means of coding pain drawings is in terms of their appropriateness. Ransford, Cairns, and Mooney (1976) developed a rating system for pain drawings based on whether they were judged to represent normal or abnormal distributions of pain. Drawings were considered normal when the distribution of pain outlined was consistent with: (a) lesions affecting the disk, spinal cord, face, or intervertebral disk, or (b) the femoral or sciatic distribution of the three common disk levels. Drawings were considered abnormal when the patient obtained 3 or more "penalty" points for: (a) unreal drawings (usually given a penalty point of 2); (b) drawings showing expansion or magnification of pain (usually given a penalty point of 1); (c) "I particularly hurt here" indicators (given a score of 1); or (d) "Look how bad I am" indicators (given a score of 1 or 2 depending on the amount of body area involved). Ransford et al. (1976) found the rating of the drawing to be closely associated with elevated Hysteria (Hs) or Hypochondriasis (Hy) scales of the Minnesota Multiphasic Personality Inventory. The Hysteria scale is designed to measure the degree to which patients are likely to somatize psychological difficulties, whereas the Hypochondriasis scale is designed to measure the willingness of individuals to endorse physical complaints. (See Chapter 4 for a more detailed discussion of the use of the MMPI with pain patients.) Unfortunately, although the relationship between abnormal pain drawings and measures of psychopathology has continued to be positive in subsequent studies, the relation has been relatively weak (cf. Schwartz & DeGood, 1984; Von Baeyer, Bergstrom, Brodwin, & Brodwin, 1983). Therefore, we do not recommend that pain drawings be used as a measure of psychopathology. Rather, they should be used to assess simply what they measure well — the location of the patient in pain and the amount of surface area involved in the pain. These measures can clearly provide the clinician with essential information on the stability of the patient's pain over time (i.e., does the pain move around and/or increase or decrease in area?) and as a function of treatment.

Chapter 4
Measures of Psychological Status

For decades, clinicians have used standardized questionnaires to assess the psychological status of pain patients. The use of these measures follows from the assumption, borne out repeatedly in the clinical and empirical literature, that the pain patient's psychological status has important implications for the planning, implementation, and outcome of treatment.

Standardized questionnaires have many advantages over other modalities of assessment. Because patients can often complete questionnaires without supervision, important information can be obtained with relatively little investment of the clinician's time. For instruments that have demonstrated their validity for use with pain patients, questionnaire results can illuminate areas of concern that might otherwise have gone unnoticed. Because questionnaires depend on self-report, they may be subject to intentional and unintentional bias and distortion. Clinicians should therefore be cautious about placing too much faith in questionnaire results, and corroborate questionnaire-based conclusions with observations and information drawn from additional sources.

Many standardized questionnaires are used in the evaluation of pain patients, indexing a variety of constructs and dimensions. The questionnaires discussed in this chapter may be classified into three overlapping categories: (a) measures of psychopathology and psychological symptoms; (b) measures of responses to pain; and (c) measures of pain-related attitudes and beliefs.

MEASURES OF PSYCHOPATHOLOGY AND PSYCHOLOGICAL SYMPTOMS

Several questionnaires are available to help assess the psychological attributes of pain patients, including the Minnesota Multiphasic Personality Inventory; the Symptom Checklist-90—Revised; the Millon Behavioral Health Inventory; the Beck Depression Inventory; the Zung Self-Rating Depression Scale; the State–Trait Anxiety Inventory; the Profile of Mood States; and the Back Pain Classification Scale.

Minnesota Multiphasic Personality Inventory

The Minnesota Multiphasic Personality Inventory (MMPI) is a 566-item true-false questionnaire designed to assess the severity of several specific psychiatric conditions. Respondents should be at least 16 years old and should have a sixth grade reading level. Although there are hundreds of scales that may be derived from the MMPI, the most commonly used include 3 validity and 10 clinical scales. Two additional scales are occasionally employed with pain patients: the Low Back Pain Scale (Lb) and the Dorsal Scale (DOR).

The validity scales were developed to assess the degree to which respondents may be: trying to present themselves in a favorable light (L or the Lie Scale), giving atypical responses, or exaggerating their difficulties, or both (F or Frequency Scale), or denying problems (K or Correction Scale). The clinical scales were designed to measure the severity of: Hypochondriasis (tendency to admit to a number of bodily complaints), Depression, Hysteria (predisposition to use conversion as a means of coping with stress), Psychopathic Deviance (history of nonconformance and antisocial behavior), Paranoia, Psychasthenia (obsessive–compulsive tendencies, or anxiety, or both), Schizophrenia, and Hypomania. However, it should be remembered that an elevated score (usually a T score greater than or equal to 70) on one of the clinical scales does not by itself establish that the patient should be diagnosed accordingly. Two additional scales, sometimes also categorized as clinical, assess Masculinity-Femininity and Social Introversion.

The MMPI is best used to assess what it was designed to assess: psychopathology. By examining the profile of scale scores, hypotheses may be entertained regarding: (a) the validity of the responses; (b) the degree of psychological distress the patient may be experiencing and how this distress may be manifesting itself (e.g., depression or anxiety); and (c) the prediction of behaviors and coping styles (cf. Lachar, 1974). The ability of trained clinicians to develop hypotheses from an MMPI profile and the existence of extensive research supporting the accuracy of many such hypotheses are probably the major reasons for the inventory's widespread use.

Several studies have examined the specific use of the MMPI with pain patients. There is some indication that the MMPI may be useful as a predictor of treatment outcome in pain patients who receive conservative treatment, surgery, pain clinic services, relaxation training, or some combination thereof. The scale most often associated with treatment outcome is the Hypochondriasis (Hs) Scale. However, inconsistent findings, such as those of Waring, Weisz, and Bailey (1976), and generally weak, although usually statistically significant, relationships between MMPI scales and treatment outcome measures suggest that clinicians should generally be cautious in using the MMPI predictively.

Studies examining the relation between MMPI subscale scores and other pain-related variables indicate that: (a) MMPI scale scores are rarely related to pain intensity; (b) elevations across the clinical scales are associated with the report of more distress and emotional discomfort as indexed by qualitative measures of pain such as the McGill Pain Questionnaire (see Chapter 3); and (c) elevations on some subscales (most often Hs and Hy, sometimes D) are associated with greater disability and functional limitation.

A promising area of study has been the identification of specific MMPI profiles among pain patients, followed by attempts to predict pain and pain-related variables as a function of these profiles. The four most common MMPI profiles thus far identified are the normal profile (T scores on all scales less than 70); the 1–3 profile (significant elevations on scales Hs and Hy); the 1–2–3 profile (significant elevations on scales Hs, D, and Hy); and the generally disturbed profile (significant elevations on Hs, D, and Hy, and an elevation on at least one, but usually more than one, other scale). A profile found less frequently is the 2 profile, identified by an elevation on the Depression Scale. Preliminary research has identified specific pain-related variables associated with profile type. Consistently, individuals with a profile indicative of greater psychopathology (e.g., the general disturbance profile) display more severe pain symptoms than do patients with a normal profile. Variables associated with disturbed MMPI profiles include pain severity, body area in pain, sleep difficulties, restriction of physical activities, and the incidence of continuous pain (Armenutrout, Moore, Parker, Hewett, & Feltz, 1982; Bradley & Van der Heide, 1984).

Preliminary research indicates that treatment outcomes may be associated with profile type. One study found that patients with at-risk profiles (i.e., elevations in one of the following combinations of scales: 123, 13, 12, 23, 18, 38, 138) were less likely to return to normal activities following conservative treatment of their chronic low back pain (McCreary, Turner, & Dawson, 1979). Profile type did not predict pain relief. Another study found that patients with at-risk profiles were less likely to return to work following treatment in a multidisciplinary pain program, although profile type was not associated with changes in mobility, activity, or treatment-seeking after therapy (Trief & Yuan, 1983). These initial findings argue for the importance of examining the entire profile response of the pain patient and the potential utility of profile analysis in predicting treatment outcome.

As already mentioned, elevations on the Hs and Hy subscales are common among pain patients as among most other chronically ill populations as well. This is not surprising, given that these scales require patients to report on the extent of their physical symptoms. Because most pain patients experience symptoms, elevations on Hs and Hy subscales among pain patients have a different meaning than do such elevations among well populations and should not be interpreted in the same way, that is, as a possible indication of the tendency to exaggerate symptoms or to convert emotional stress into physical complaints.

Despite the many attempts to find or develop MMPI scales that discriminate organic from functional pain patients, no scale, including the Lb and DOR subscales, which were both designed specifically to identify functional patients, has been able to consistently differentiate among pain patients with a clear organic cause and patients whose pain has no currently measurable origin. Therefore, the use of the MMPI in diagnosing a patient's pain as functional or organic should be considered highly questionable.

Because research on the use of the MMPI with pain patients is in its nascent stages relative to research on the MMPI psychiatric patients, clinicians must depend on their clinical experience to interpret the profiles. Fordyce (1979), in a monograph describing the use of the MMPI with pain patients, provides several recommendations based on his extensive experience with both the MMPI and patients with chronic pain. He found that the MMPI may be used to: rule out depression as a diagnosis when the complaint is pain; examine cognitive deficits that may be associated with narcotic drug use; rule out cortical deficits; examine indications of tension states; and predict the patient's readiness to use pain to manipulate others. Guidelines for employing the MMPI to address these questions are provided in Fordyce's monograph. Although some of his recommendations have yet to undergo adequate empirical examination, they represent an important and helpful source of ideas when using the MMPI in the assessment of pain patients.

One common criticism of the MMPI is its length. Pain patients can take from 1 to 3 hours to fill out the inventory. To justify its use, clinicians should be able to answer yes to two questions: (a) Is the MMPI capable of providing a valid answer to a specific question about this pain patient? and (b) Is there no other scale or procedure capable of answering the question that is as useful, but less time-consuming than the MMPI?

Symptom Checklist-90—Revised

The Symptom Checklist-90—Revised (SCL-90—R; Derogatis, 1977) is designed to assess psychological symptom patterns. Responders are asked to indicate how much they have been bothered by 90 specific symptoms on a 5-point scale ranging from not at all to extremely. The 90 symptom descriptions are classified into 9 symptom dimensions: somatization, obsessive-compulsive, interpersonal sensitivity, depression, anxiety, hostility, phobic anxiety, paranoid ideation, and psychoticism. The SCL-90—R may be scored to yield measures on the 9 dimensions and can also provide three general measures of distress: global severity index, positive symptom distress index, and positive symptom total. Although originally developed as a criterion measure in psychotherapeutic drug trials, the scale is now being employed in multiple settings to gauge psychological symptoms.

The SCL-90—R demonstrates adequate internal consistency and test-retest stability for all of the nine dimensions and three global scores. The major limitation of the scale appears to be the lack of discriminability between its 9 dimensions, that is, the scale scores are highly intercorrelated (cf. Gotlib, 1984).

Little research has been performed using the SCL-90—R among pain patients. Therefore, its use as a measure in this population is difficult to judge. In one study of chronic pain patients, the construct validity of the anxiety and depression subscales was revealed by their significant correlation to other, more established measures of these constructs (Duckro, Margolis, & Tait, 1985). However, a high degree of interscale correlation was again in evidence, suggesting that the subscales of the SCL-90—R reflect general distress rather than 9 distinct symptom dimensions. These results indicate that until further evidence proves otherwise, pain assessors can place confidence only in the depression subscale scores, anxiety subscale score, and global severity index of the SCL-90—R.

Millon Behavioral Health Inventory

The Millon Behavioral Inventory (MBHI; Millon, Green, & Meagher, 1979) is a 150-item self-report questionnaire designed to be used in medical settings. The inventory contains 20 subscales, 8 to assess personality styles that are hypothesized to predict how a person might develop and cope with disease; 6 to measure psychogenic attitudes believed to be associated with the course of physical illness; 3 psychosomatic correlates designed to predict a patient's tendency to develop specific illness; and 3 prognostic indices to appraise emotional factors believed to complicate ailments or predict psychological complications associated with specific diseases. One prognostic index, the Pain Treatment Responsivity Scale PP, is designed specifically to be used with pain patients. This scale is made up of items that were found to discriminate between patients who demonstrated a successful response to medical treatment for pain and patients who proved unresponsive to treatment.

There is a need for a questionnaire that can do what the MBHI was designed to do, that is, to provide measures of attitudes and traits that influence the course of the disease and provide indications for appropriate treatments. However, it is unclear that the MBHI fulfils this purpose. Over the 8 years since the scale was introduced, there have been few published reports of the inventory's validity. One group of investigators found that no MBHI subscale was associated with pain-related variables such as the number of hospitalizations, number of pain medications, and duration of pain (Sweet, Breuer, Hazlewood, Toye, & Pawl, 1985). Only one scale (Introversion) demonstrated a small but statistically significant relationship to the number of pain operations. Regarding the ability of the MBHI to predict treatment outcome in a multidisciplinary pain treatment program, Sweet et al. (1985) found that (a) the PP scale predicted treatment outcome less well than did other scales of the MBHI, (b) the PP scale had only a 70% accuracy rate for discriminating successful from unsuccessful outcomes, and (c) the PP scale was closely associated with 10 of the other MBHI scales, indicating that the PP scale lacks specificity.

Another study found that a good prognosis prediction (based on the MBHI) to traditional outpatient treatment was actually associated with an increased number of pain-related hospitalizations following treatment on a neurosurgery ward (Murphy, Sperr, & Sperr, 1986). In a third study, 11 MBHI scales were significantly associated with changes in the number of headaches following behavioral treatment for headache pain, 4 were associated with decreases in headache duration, 1 scale predicted decreases in medication use, and no scale was associated with changes in pain intensity (Gatchel, Deckel, Weinberg, & Smith, 1985). However, because of the small sample size and the exploratory nature (i.e., many analyses were performed) of this third study, the results obtained should be considered as preliminary.

Although the MBHI is purportedly designed for use with medical populations, it has thus far performed no better than the MMPI in predicting treatment outcome. The amount of validity research performed to date provides mixed results for the use of the MBHI with pain patients. Clearly, additional validity research with the MBHI will be necessary before the inventory can be recommended for use in the assessment of pain patients.

Pain and Depression

The three measures of depression used most often with pain patients are the Beck Depression Inventory (BDI; Beck, Rush, Shaw, & Emery, 1979), the Zung Self-Rating Depression Scale (Zung, 1965), and the depression scale of the Minnesota Multiphasic Personality Inventory. Both the BDI and the Zung scale are brief (21 and 20 items, respectively), self-administered questionnaires that require the patient to report on the incidence of various symptoms of depression. In a recent study, the BDI and the Zung scale demonstrated good sensitivity and specificity in their ability to classify depressed and nondepressed chronic pain patients, and both performed better than the depression scale of the MMPI (Turner & Romano, 1984). These results argue for the use of one of these scales when assessing pain patients in whom depression is a concern, even when the MMPI is administered.

Additional evidence for the usefulness of measuring depression in chronic pain patients has been presented by Keefe, Wilkins, Cook, Crisson, and Muhlbaier (in press), who found meaningful variables such as pain intensity, overt pain behavior, activity level, and medication intake to all be associated with depression as measured by the BDI, controlling for demographic and medical status variables. In addition, the BDI has been a useful predictor of response to relaxation training among pain patients (Jacob, Turner, Szekely, & Eidelman, 1983).

One possible criticism of both the BDI and the Zung scale is that they include items that deal with physical symptoms. Because many chronic pain patients are likely to have genuine physical problems, they might tend to score higher on depression inventories even if they have no other symptoms of depression. However, at least for the BDI, depression scores do not appear to be confounded by organic pathology (Crisson, Keefe, Wilkins, Cook, & Muhlbaier, 1986). Because of the high incidence of depression in chronic pain patients, we recommend that it be routinely checked for and the BDI and Zung scale appear to be the most useful means.

State–Trait Anxiety Inventory

Anxiety is another emotion commonly associated with pain. In fact, anxiety has so much in common with pain in terms of how it is measured, how persons respond physiologically, and how it is treated (cf. Gross & Collins, 1981), that it can be difficult at times to distinguish one from the other.

The most common measure of the anxiety construct among pain patients is the State–Trait Anxiety Inventory (STAI; Spielberger, 1983). This 40-item inventory measures two kinds of anxiety: trait anxiety, which is ". . . the tendency to perceive stressful situations as dangerous or threatening and to respond to such situations with elevations in the intensity of their state anxiety . . ." (Spielberger, 1983, p. 1), and state anxiety, which is the level of anxiety experienced at a specific time, usually in response to a specific situation. Patients are asked to respond to 20 feeling statements with respect to how they feel right now (state anxiety) and how they feel generally (trait anxiety). The reliability and construct validity of both the old (Form X) and new (Form Y) versions of the STAI are excellent.

Despite the theoretical importance of anxiety in the experience of pain, few studies have examined the use of anxiety measures with pain patients. In one of these studies, neither subscale of the STAI was associated with pain duration in facial pain patients, but both demonstrated a small but significant relationship to pain intensity (Marbach & Lund, 1981). In another study, trait anxiety was associated with chronicity of pain, whereas state anxiety was not (Garron & Leavitt, 1983). In a third experiment, state anxiety demonstrated a weak (but statistically significant) relationship to pain intensity, while trait anxiety was not associated with intensity measures. In addition, in a group of low back pain patients, the anxiety scales demonstrated very weak (mostly nonsignificant) relationships to subscales of the Low Back Questionnaire, which measures various qualitative aspects of the pain experience (Garron & Leavitt, 1979).

In sum, although the STAI is known to be a valid measure of state and trait anxiety, and anxiety has been hypothesized to be an important variable in pain patients, evidence published to date indicates that anxiety measures are not strongly associated with other constructs often measured in pain patients and so may not be a useful predictor of these other variables. The STAI may nonetheless be useful as a supplemental treatment outcome measure.

Profile of Mood States

Pain has been hypothesized to influence and be influenced by general mood states. Accordingly, some investigators have explored the relation between validated measures of mood and various pain-related constructs. The mood measure employed most often has been the Profile of Mood States (POMS; McNair, Lorr, & Droppleman, 1971). Research generally has found that pain intensity correlates weakly but positively with negative mood (cf. Shacham, Reinhardt, Raubertas, & Cleeland, 1983). However, research that examines the relationship between mood measures and other important components of pain has yet to be performed. Therefore, it is not clear that measuring mood is clinically useful in understanding the chronic pain patient, especially over and above the use of other measures of affect.

Back Pain Classification Scale

The Back Pain Classification Scale (BPCS; Leavitt & Garron, 1979b) was designed to assess the contribution of psychological factors to a patient's pain. It was constructed by selecting 13 pain descriptors from the Low Back Pain Questionnaire (see Chapter 3), which discriminated low back pain patients who had clear signs of organic disease from patients who had minimal or no organic signs and who were judged to have "significant emotional disturbance". Although problems with the original criterion groups, most notably the confounding between the level of organicity and the level of psychological disturbance, are evident, high scores on the BPCS have been associated with elevations on all clinical scales of the MMPI (Leavitt & Garron, 1980). However, even though it is recommended that the scale be used as a screening device for general psychological disturbance and the high scores be used to indicate the necessity of a full psychological evaluation (Leavitt, 1983), a series of studies examining the accuracy rate of the Low Back Pain Questionnaire for identifying chronic pain patients with psychological disturbance should be performed before its use as a screening device can be recommended.

MEASURES OF RESPONSES TO PAIN

Another subset of standardized questionnaires has been designed to assess the effects of chronic pain on the lives of pain patients. How does pain interfere with day-to-day functioning? How is the patient coping with pain? How are family members dealing with the patient's problems? Instruments designed to tap ecologically meaningful reactions to pain can assist clinicians in understanding the severity of the pain problem in the "big picture" of the patient's daily functioning (a Context II concern) and can help in evaluating treatments designed to decrease pain's negative life impact. The scales that fall into this category assess a variety of responses including the impact of pain on day-to-day activities (the Health Assessment Questionnaire and the Sickness Impact Profile); pain coping strategies (Coping Strategy Questionnaire; Vanderbilt Pain Management Inventory); assertiveness skills (Rathus Assertiveness Scale); and a multidimensional measure of responses to pain (the West-Haven Yale Multidimensional Pain Inventory).

Health Assessment Questionnaire

The Health Assessment Questionnaire (HAQ; Fries, Spitz, & Young, 1982) was designed to be an index of health treatment outcome. The questionnaire is extensive and assesses four dimensions: disability, pain, drug side effects, and health care costs. The most recent version of the disability subscale consists of 20 items that require patients to indicate on 4-point scale how able they are to perform routine daily activities. To measure pain, the HAQ employs a Visual Analogue Scale (see Chapter 3). The remainder of the questionnaire consists of 15 pages of questions that inquire specifically about drug use, drug side effects, treatments obtained, and treatment costs.

The disability scale of the HAQ has received the most research attention. It has demonstrated adequate to excellent construct and convergent validity (Fries, Spitz, Kraines, & Holman, 1980). These results argue for the inclusion of the disability subscale in any comprehensive test battery.

Sickness Impact Profile

The Sickness Impact Profile (SIP; Bergner, Bobbitt, Carter, & Gilson, 1981) is a 136-item behaviorally based measure of health status. The SIP covers 12 categories of activity involved in normal living including ambulation, mobility, body care and movement, social interaction, communication, alertness behavior, emotional behavior, sleep and rest, eating, work, home management, and recreation and pastimes. Scoring the SIP yields measures for each of the 12 categories, a measure of 2 dimensions of health status (physical and psychosocial dimensions) and an overall disability score. The SIP can be self-administered or administered by an interviewer, whereas mail-delivered SIPs appear unable to provide data comparable to interview- or self-administered responses (Bergner et al., 1981). Test-retest and internal consistency coefficients are excellent for the overall SIP score. Also, evidence supports the adequacy of the construct, convergent, and discriminant validity of SIP's 12 dimensions (Bergner et al., 1981).

Recently, the use of the SIP was examined in chronic low back pain patients referred to a multidisciplinary chronic pain treatment program (Follick, Smith, & Ahern, 1985). The results support the construct and discriminant validity of the SIP and indicate that the scale is sensitive enough to detect pre- to post-treatment changes. The authors conclude that the SIP

appears extremely well suited in terms of reliability, validity, breadth of assessment and ease of administration, for the assessment of patients suffering from chronic pain and as an instrument for evaluating the efficacy of multi-disciplinary pain clinics (Follick et al., 1985, p. 75).

Based on the evidence, we agree that the SIP is an excellent measure for assessing changes in the functioning of pain patients in response to treatments or over time, especially if a more detailed analysis of functioning than that obtained with the HAQ is desired.

MEASURES OF PAIN COPING

To treat pain, the clinician needs to understand what specific coping strategies the patient is currently employing and the effectiveness of these strategies. Some of this information can be obtained during the clinical interview (see Chapter 7). However, two promising paper-and-pencil measures of general pain-coping strategies are currently being developed.

One instrument is the Coping Strategy Questionnaire (CSQ; Rosenstiel & Keefe, 1983). It was designed to assess the degree to which patients employ six separate cognitive strategies (diverting attention, reinterpreting pain sensations, using coping self-statements, ignoring pain sensations, praying or hoping, and catastrophizing) and a single behavioral coping strategy (increasing activity level). Six items provide data on each strategy. In addition, the scale contains two questions that require patients to indicate how much control they feel they have over pain and how able they are to decrease pain. Patients respond to all items along a 7-point scale. The seven scale scores and two effectiveness ratings have been combined, through factor analysis, into three general coping measures: Cognitive Coping and Suppression (CCS), Helplessness, and Diverting Attention and Praying (DAP). Unfortunately, individual item analyses have not been performed, such that items of poor quality may remain in the scale. In addition, cross-validation of the original factor analysis has not yet been performed. The lack of published internal consistency and test-retest stability coefficients for the general measures of coping makes it difficult to judge the reliability of these measures. However, intercorrelations between the general measures, although moderate in two cases, are low enough to suggest that the different measures indeed assess different aspects of coping.

Despite the scale's psychometric limitations, the three general measures of coping have been predictive of other pain-related variables. The DAP scores demonstrate a moderate relationship to pain intensity ($r=0.59$) and the degree to which pain interferes with daily activities ($r=0.53$). Less impressive relationships were found between the CCS measure and pain intensity ($r=0.21$), depression ($r=0.27$), anxiety ($r=0.27$), and interference with daily activities ($r=0.18$). Finally, the Helplessness measure was somewhat predictive of depression (as measured by the Zung scale, $r=0.38$) and of anxiety ($r=0.34$) (Rosenstiel & Keefe, 1983). In another study, the DAP and Helplessness measures predicted surgical response 41 days after treatment in a group of patients who underwent lumbar laminectomy (Gross, 1986). These results argue for the potential importance of assessing general coping efforts among pain patients. However, further development of the CSQ (i.e., item analyses and cross-validation of the original factor analysis) is indicated before the scale can be highly recommended for use in clinical settings. In addition, judging from the direction of many of the correlations already described, the CSQ may be best thought of as an index of coping effort rather than coping success.

A second general coping questionnaire still in its early stages of development is the Vanderbilt Pain Management Inventory (VPMI; Brown & Nicassio, 1985). This 21-item questionnaire contains questions designed to assess the frequency with which pain patients employ active and passive cognitive and behavioral pain-coping strategies. Careful scale development has resulted in a two-dimension questionnaire that appears to have adequate reliability and construct validity. Although additional research examining the use of the VPMI has yet to be performed, preliminary evidence and the strong psychometric properties of the scale suggest that the VPMI may be useful in identifying the coping activities of pain patients.

Rathus Assertiveness Scale

Many multidisciplinary pain programs teach assertiveness skills under the assumption that increased assertiveness among chronic pain patients will increase their communication skills with family and friends, thereby enabling them to achieve interpersonal goals. Accordingly, a brief questionnaire is needed to indicate who might benefit from assertiveness training as well as to assess treatment outcome.

The most commonly used measure of assertiveness is the Rathus Assertiveness Scale (RAS; Ruthus, 1973), a 30-item instrument that has demonstrated adequate internal consistency and predictive validity (predicting assertive behaviors). As an outcome measure in a treatment evaluation study of a multidisciplinary pain program, the scale has demonstrated sensitivity to treatment effects (Block, Kremer, & Gaylor, 1980a). In short, the scale appears to be an adequate brief measure of assertiveness that may be employed with pain patients.

West Haven-Yale Multidimensional Pain Inventory

The West Haven-Yale Multidimensional Pain Inventory (WHYMPI; Kerns, Turk, & Rudy, 1985) was designed to provide a comprehensive assessment of the "subjective experience of pain". The questionnaire has three sections. The first consists of five subscales that assess: (a) the perceived interference of pain in daily activities; (b) the support patients experience from significant others (e.g., spouse); (c) pain severity; (d) perceived self-control over life and life's problems; and (e) negative mood. The second section measures three responses that the patient perceives from his or her significant other: (a) punishing responses; (b) solicitous responses; and (c) distracting responses. Finally, the third section seeks to tap the frequency with which the patient participates in four categories of activity: (a) household chores; (b) outdoor work; (d) activities away from home; and (d) social activities.

The WHYMPI subscales have all demonstrated adequate internal consistency and test-retest stability. A lack of association between subscales suggests that each subscale measures something unique. Preliminary evidence for the validity of the scales is provided in the initial published report, although more research is needed to provide evidence for the specific meanings of the subscales and to indicate what other pain variables may be predicted from WHYMPI subscale scores. Mainly because of the careful development of the WHYMPI, the scale holds promise as a measure of various important aspects of the pain experience which have not yet been assessed by other instruments.

MEASURES OF PAIN-RELATED ATTITUDES AND BELIEFS

The final category of standardized questionnaires to be discussed in this chapter are measures of attitudes and beliefs about pain. Two scales that assess such constructs are the Illness Behavior Questionnaire and the Health Index.

Illness Behavior Questionnaire

The most recently revised Illness Behavior Questionnaire (IBQ; Pilowsky, Spence, Cobb, & Katsikitis, 1984) is a 62-item self-administered inventory designed to be a multicomponent measure of the way persons "experience and respond to their health status". Forty of the items can be scored to yield seven specific attitudes and beliefs about health (Scale 1: General Hypochondriasis; Scale 2: Disease Conviction; Scale 3: Psychologic versus Somatic Perception of Illness; Scale 4: Affective Inhibition; Scale 5: Affective Disturbances; Scale 6: Denial; Scale 7: Irritability), two factor scales (Disease Affirmation, made up of scales 2 and 3, and Affective State made up of scales 1, 5, and 7), a scale consisting of items that discriminate between patients attending a pain clinic and patients attending a general practitioner's surgery (called the Conversion Scale on the assumption that pain clinic patients displayed more conversion symptoms), and the Whitely Index of Hypochrondriasis, which consists of items that discriminate between psychiatric patients who had been diagnosed as manifesting hypochondriacal features and psychiatric patients who demonstrated little or no evidence of hypochondriasis (Pilowsky, 1967).

Despite the potential use of the IBQ, methodological problems were associated with the procedures employed to develop the instrument. Most significantly, the number of subjects who participated in the original scale development was too small for adequate item analysis or the development of specific subscales. As a result, no subsequent study has found the same dimensions as the original, suggesting that the seven original subscales need refinement. One study, which did employ an adequate number of subjects, found that all of the subscales correlated highly with measures of neuroticism (i.e., general affective disturbance), whereas another study found that six of the seven IBQ scales demonstrated a substantial relationship to the MMPI Depression scale (Stein, Fruchter, & Trief, 1983). The lack of stability of factors and the strong relationship between IBQ scales and measures of emotional discomfort suggest that the IBQ lacks discriminant validity.

Despite the psychometric problems with the IBQ, several studies do indicate that the instrument is related to some important pain-related variables. For example, subscales of the IBQ differentially predict specific pain behaviors (Keefe, Crisson, Maltbie, Bradley, & Gil, in press). *Disease Conviction* predicted the tendency to rub painful areas; *Affective Inhibition* predicted the use of devices (e.g., canes, walkers, and furniture) during movement and when static; *Affective Disturbance* predicted the use of devices when static; *Denial* predicted limping; and the *Psychologic-Somatic* subscale predicted sighing. Regarding the prediction of the qualitative aspects of pain as measured by the McGill Pain Questionnaire, *Irritability* predicted scores on the sensory dimension, and both Denial and Irritability were associated with the evaluative dimension of pain. Undoubtedly, the potential utility of the scale will be greatly enhanced when efforts are made to improve its psychometric properties.

Health Index

The Health Index (Sternbach, Wolf, Murphy, & Akeson, 1973) is a 50-item, yes–no format questionnaire designed to assess the psychological factors of pain. The index has four subscales. First is the Invalidism scale, which assesses the degree to which the patient has dropped out of life as a result of pain. Nine of the 10 items on this scale came from the Cornell Medical Index (Brodman, Erdmann, Lorge, & Wolff, 1949). The second scale consists of the 20 items from the Zung Self-Rating Depression Scale (Zung, 1965). The third and fourth scales were designed to assess, respectively, the impact of pain on the patients' lives and the degree to which patients participate in pain game playing.

Although the Health Index demonstrated diagnostic sensitivity by differentiating arthritis from low back pain patients, no research has since been performed to cross-validate the initial promising findings and to provide further evidence of validity. In addition, reliability estimates, that is, internal consistency and test-retest stability measures, have not been published for this scale. Therefore, until the scale's psychometric properties are better known, we recommend that little emphasis be placed on the individual scale scores. However, because the questionnaire does inquire about attitudes not assessed by other questionnaires, especially the items on the game-playing subscale, individual item responses may be used to identify potential areas for further inquiry. For example, responses to certain subscale items may indicate that the patient is feeling frustrated about the way he or she has been treated in the past by members of the medical profession. (*Note*: Such feelings are not necessarily evidence for game playing, because some medical personnel have not been adequately trained to treat chronic pain patients.) Negative attitudes may color the patient's current interactions with treatment providers and interfere with the treatment course. Therefore, through assessment of and subsequent intervention in specific counter-therapeutic attitudes, clinicians may be able to short-circuit potential treatment difficulties.

Chapter 5
Biophysical Measurement

The anatomy and physiology of pain are both highly complex, and our knowledge of this complexity has been accumulating at a rapid pace over the last two decades. Concurrent with this increase in knowledge has been the development of increasingly sophisticated physiological pain-assessment methods. Although some biophysical procedures have demonstrated clinical relevance, many need further study and development before their utility in the assessment of clinical pain can be adequately judged. In this chapter, some promising biophysical measures of pain will be briefly described and critiqued. The measurement techniques covered include percutaneous neurography, biochemical activity measurement, evoked potentials, electromyography, and the assessment of autonomic responses.

PERCUTANEOUS NEUROGRAPHY

Percutaneous neurography, a relatively recent development, is a method for measuring the activity in nerve fibers that transmit pain messages from the periphery, that is, areas of the body outside of the central nervous system, to the spine. Pain-transmitting fibers are found in densely packed bundles within the limbs. The nociceptive fibers within these bundles vary in diameter and include the thick, myelinated A-delta fibers and the thin, unmyelinated C fibers.

In percutaneous neurography, an epoxy-coated (except for the tip) tungsten wire is inserted through the skin into a bundle of afferent nerve fibers. The electrical activity of the fibers is then measured and recorded.

Most often, percutaneous neurography has been used to assess nerve activity in response to laboratory pain, consistently demonstrating that painful stimuli and the report of pain sensations are accompanied by increases in neural activity of the A-delta and C fibers (cf. Vallbo, Hagbarth, Torebjork, & Wallin, 1979). Although not much research has explored neurography as an index of clinical pain, research to date has demonstrated that the technique can provide useful data on nerve activity in chronic pain states, such as phantom limb pain

(Nystrom & Hagbarth, 1981) and causalgia (Wallin, Torebjork, & Hallin, 1976).

Unfortunately, the use of percutaneous neurography involves some negative effects and risks. First, when the nerve bundle is impaled, the subject usually experiences some pain and paresthesia (an uncomfortable tingling or numbing sensation). Also, some subjects may experience prolonged tenderness at the site of exploration. Hallin (1984) reports that in no case among hundreds has permanent nerve damage resulted, although he does caution that percutaneous neurography has a potential risk of nerve damage and should be used with caution.

In sum, percutaneous neurography has demonstrated its use in the assessment of nociceptive neural impulses reaching the spinal cord. The positive findings from studies using the procedure to study causalgia and phantom limb pain support additional research to extend the use of the method in the assessment of clinical pain states.

BIOCHEMICAL ASSESSMENT

One of the most exciting advances in pain research over the last decade has been the increased understanding of inherent, or endogenous, pain-control systems. Strong evidence now exists that at the point at which pain impulses enter the spinal cord, they can be subjected to inhibitory influences from higher centers of the brain. At least one pain inhibition system involves the release of endogenous morphine-like substances, called endorphins, from neurons in the midbrain. Once released, endorphins bind to specific receptors on other neurons to initiate the transmission of pain-inhibitory signals, which eventually reach the spinal cord and act to decrease or close the gate on incoming pain signals from the periphery. By measuring the activity of endorphins, indirect assessment can be obtained of the degree of activity of the descending (centrifugal) pain suppression system. Although we shall emphasize the form of endogenous pain supression based on morphine-like or opioid paths, it should be noted that nonopioid forms of pain control also exist (Lewis, Nelson, Terman, Shavit, & Liebeskind, 1986).

Two methods have been used to measure endorphin activity. One involves the administration of a chemical that blocks the activity of some endorphins, and the other involves the direct measurement of the level of endorphins in body fluids.

In the endorphin-blocking method, naloxone is used as the endorphin antagonist (blocking agent). Once naloxone is injected intravenously, it locks onto neurotransmitter receptors, such as those in the midbrain, used by some endorphins. This effectively blocks endorphins from using these receptors to facilitate a pain-inhibition signal. If a patient's report of pain increases more than would be expected following the administration of naloxone, then the endorphin-modulated pain suppression system is likely to have been active in that patient.

As should be clear, the endorphin-blocking method is especially useful for assessing the current activity of the endorphin-modulated pain inhibition system, and therefore can be used to assess the degree to which a particular treatment operates through this system. Also, naloxone can be used to assess the regular activity of this system in clinical pain states. Naloxone injections have been used to support the importance of the endorphin system in accounting for the analgesic properties of some kinds of acupuncture, transcutaneous nerve stimulation, placebo analgesia, and stimulation-produced analgesia (cf. Watkins & Mayer, 1982). Also, injections of naloxone in chronic pain patients have not changed their reported pain experience, suggesting that the endorphin pain inhibition system is not usually operating in these patients (Lindblom & Tegner, 1979).

The second method of assessing endorphin activity involves the collection of some body fluid and the measurement, through biochemical analyses, of the amount of endorphins in that fluid. Measures of endorphin levels are usually made in cerebrospinal fluid (CSF) because endorphin activity within the central nervous system is of greatest interest. Other body fluids, such as blood plasma or urine, tend to be used less often because of their greater distance from the central nervous system. In employing biochemical measures of endorphin levels, it is assumed that the higher the level of endorphins found, the greater the endorphin activity.

Measuring endorphin levels in CSF is not without problems. First, CSF is usually collected through lumbar puncture, or spinal tap, which in itself is a painful experience. Second, there is no solid evidence that the CSF endorphin level, taken from the lumbar region, reflects the level at other sites in the nervous system. In fact, the results of one study suggest that the endorphin level assessed may indeed be influenced by the site of CSF collection (Sjölund, Terenius, & Eriksson, 1977). Finally, it is not clear which members of the endorphin family are being measured by the currently used biochemical techniques. Many different endorphins are known to exist, each belonging to one of three peptide families (Akil, Watson, Young, Lewis, Khatchurian, & Walker, 1984). Currently used measurement strategies, although able to identify compounds as being much like endorphins, cannot always identify which specific types are being measured (Terenius, 1984). Therefore, the relative importance of some endorphins has yet to be thoroughly determined.

Despite the problems involved in measuring endorphin levels, research using endorphin level measurement techniques have yielded important and interesting findings. First, various treatments have been associated with increases of endorphins in the CSF or blood plasma, including stimulation-produced analgesia (Akil, Richardson, Hughes, & Barchas, 1978; Hosobuchi,

Rossier, Bloom, & Guillemin, 1979), electro-acupuncture (Sjölund, Terenius, & Eriksson, 1977), and acupuncture (Kiser, Gatchel, Bhatia, Khatami, Huang, & Altchuler, 1983).

In addition, studies have shown endorphin levels to be associated with some chronic pain states. Chronic pain and headache patients possess a lower endorphin level than do normal subjects (Akil, Richardson, Hughes, & Barchas, 1978; Sicuteri, Anselmi, Curradi, Michelacci, & Sassi, 1978; Terenius & Wahlström, 1975). In another study, patients diagnosed as having "organic" (localized) pain had significantly lower levels of CSF endorphins than patients diagnosed as having "psychogenic" (vague and nonlocalized) pain (Almay, Johansson, VonKnorring, Terenius, & Wahlström, 1978). Cleeland, Shacham, Dahl, and Orrison (1984) found CSF beta-endorphins to be negatively correlated to self-reports of pain intensity in 24 patients suspected of having vertebral disk disease, whereas Genazzani et al. (1984) found CSF beta-endorphin levels to be negatively related to the severity of impairment in migraine sufferers. These studies suggest that some chronic pain states may be related to reduced activity in the endorphin-mediated endogenous pain-suppression system.

The literature on endorphin activity in chronic pain patients strongly indicates that an important relation exists between the activity of the endorphin-modulated pain inhibition system and clinically relevant findings, such as pain level and diagnosis. Measuring this activity directly, through biochemical analyses, or indirectly, through the use of naloxone, enables an assessment of the degree to which the endorphin analyses can be helpful, not only in understanding the effectiveness of a particular patient's pain-modulating system, but also in prescribing appropriate treatments (e.g., treatments that make use of the endorphin pain inhibition system) and in assessing the effectiveness of those treatments.

EVOKED POTENTIAL MEASUREMENT

Evoked potentials (EPs) are indices of the brain's electrical response to an induced, discrete stimulus as measured from electrodes placed on the scalp. Because the brain is always active, it becomes difficult to separate general brain activity from the specific activity caused by the stimulus. This problem is overcome by averaging the brain's response to the stimulus, which is presented repeatedly, allowing the stimulus-produced response to be enhanced and the background electrical activity to be averaged out. With the proper equipment and with adequate calibration of the stimulation generator and recording devices, EPs can be relatively easily obtained (Chudler & Dong, 1983).

Evoked potentials have been studied primarily as correlates of induced experimental pain. Evidence generally indicates that the EP waveform has several components and that some late-occurring components may be closely related to the subjective perception of pain, as compared with the earlier components that correlate more strongly with the objective intensity (amount of stimulation) of the laboratory stimulus (Chapman, Chen, & Harkins, 1979; Chen, Chapman, & Harkins, 1979). The early components are sometimes labeled exogenous, representing an evoked obligatory response to sensory input. Conversely, endogenous components have been found to vary with psychological, contextual factors (Donchin, McCarthy, Kutas, & Ritter, 1983). Because the endogenous components of the EP waveform appear too late to be a direct result of A-delta fiber transmissions and too early to reflect the slow conducting C fiber impulses, these components of the EP are believed to be indices of the secondary perceptual processes associated with the experience of pain.

Although EPs have demonstrated validity as correlates of laboratory pain, they show less promise for indexing clinical pain, because the onset and degree of clinical pain cannot be closely controlled. However, one potential use of EPs in chronic pain was proposed by Chen, Treede, and Bromm (1984), who suggested that chronic pain may be measured indirectly by comparing the EPs of pain patients with the EPs of normal subjects. To the extent that chronic pain alters an individual's perception of other stimuli or in some other way decreases the perception of discrete painful stimuli, relative decreases in EPs in response to induced pain would be expected in chronic pain patients when compared with normal subjects. In a preliminary study, Chen, Treede, and Broom (1984) found both intensity ratings and EPs, in response to discrete pain, to be diminished in subjects experiencing a tonic ischemic pain (a laboratory-induced pain believed to be similar to the sensations of chronic pain) as compared with subjects not experiencing ischemic pain. This finding provided the authors with preliminary hope that EPs might be a useful index of chronic pain. However, because experimentally induced ischemic pain is not equivalent to clinical pain, additional research is needed before strong support can be claimed for the method.

ELECTROMYOGRAPHY

In electromyography (EMG), electrodes are placed on the surface of the skin just above various muscle groups. These electrodes are used to measure the small amounts of electrical activity that are produced by muscles when they are active (that is, tense). Electromyography therefore has the potential to be useful in the assessment of pain conditions that are or may be associated with abnormal muscle responses. Pain disorders studied with EMG include back pain, headache, and the myofacial pain dysfunction (MPD) syndrome.

Electromyography and Back Pain

One of the most promising uses of EMG in assessing pain is electromyographic scanning (Cram & Steger, 1983; Hoyt et al., 1981; Wolf & Basmajian, 1978). This method involves measuring and comparing muscle activity in the different muscle groups of a single pain patient. In this way, not only can overall levels of muscle activity at different sites be assessed, but also patterns of muscle activity that may be important in the pathogenesis of pain can be examined also. Three electromyographic scanning protocols have been described.

The assessment protocol of Cram and Steger (1983) consists of measuring the activity of 11 muscle groups separately on both sides of the body. In addition, the 22 sites are monitored while the patient is both sitting and standing, bringing the total number of measurements to 44. Five muscle groups are measured in the head and neck (frontalis, temporalis, masseter, sternocleidomastoid, and cervical paraspinals), five in the back (trapezius, thoracic 1 paraspinals, thoracic 6 paraspinals, thoracic 10 paraspinals, and lumbar 3 paraspinals), and one group in the abdomen (abdominals).

To assess the activity in all these muscle groups efficiently, Cram and Steger (1983) use electrodes that are mounted on posts approximately 2 cm apart. The scanning electrodes are first dipped into electrode paste, and held motionless over the site until the electromyograph yields a stable recording for over 4 seconds. It takes approximately 20 minutes to complete their protocol.

In comparing the protocols of four chronic pain populations (headache only, neck, shoulder, and upper back pain only, low back pain only, and mixed), Cram and Steger (1983) found important differences among the patients. They generally found higher levels of head muscle (frontalis and masseter) activity in the headache patients, and a trend for the low back pain patients to have a greater discrepancy between the activity of muscles measured on one side of the body versus that on the other side for the cervical paraspinals and lumbar 3 paraspinals. These findings provide preliminary validation of their procedure in the prediction of abnormal muscle activity among pain patients.

Wolf and Basmajian (1978) introduced an electromyographic protocol designed primarily for back pain patients. They assessed the right and left aspects of lumbar muscle groups. Four electrodes were placed on the lower back 3 cm from the posterior midline between the third and fourth and the fourth and fifth lumbar vertebrae. The electrodes were then used to measure electromyographic activity from the sites in four combinations: the fourth and fifth lumbar vertebrae bilaterally, the right side only (the fourth and fifth and third and fourth lumbar vertebrae), the second and fourth vertebrae bilaterally, and the left side only (the fourth and fifth and third and fourth lumbar vertebrae). In addition, electromyographic activity can be measured both while the patient is sitting quietly and while performing movements. Using this protocol to compare low back pain patients with normal subjects,

Wolf, Basmajian, Russe, and Kutner (1979) found normal subjects to consistently demonstrate symmetrical electromyographic activity when comparing left and right lumbar muscle groups during trunk flexion and extension (while the patient bends at the waist and straightens up again). However, chronic back pain patients showed asymmetrical electromyographic levels during trunk extension and flexion (Wolf, Nacht, & Kelly, 1982).

Hoyt et al. (1981) describe a third protocol in which electromyographic levels of four sites are measured simultaneously while a patient is in three positions. In the Hoyt et al. (1981) protocol, electrodes are placed on the right and left aspects of the abdominals and the fourth lumbar paraspinals. Simultaneous measures are made while the subject spends 10 minutes in each of three positions: semi-Fowler, sitting, and standing. Hoyt et al. (1981) found that only during standing was there a significant difference in electromyographic activity between chronic back pain patients and normal subjects. Specifically, during standing, the overall electromyographic activity of the fourth lumbar paraspinals was greater among pain patients than among normal subjects, and a significant difference in asymmetry was found between the left and right aspects of the paraspinals, with chronic pain patients showing a greater left-to right discrepancy. No significant difference between groups was found in the electromyographic activity of the abdominal muscles.

As a group, studies examining electromyographic activity in back pain patients show promise. Most studies support the conclusion that back pain patients have greater asymmetry than do normal subjects. Also , as suggested by both Wolf, Nacht, and Kelly (1982) and Cram and Steger (1983), electromyographic scanning can help biofeedback clinicians identify abnormal (i.e., overly active or asymmetrical electromyographic) activity, and thus pinpoint where a treatment focus may be most beneficial.

Unanswered questions include: the importance of measuring more (as in Cram and Steger's (1983) protocol) versus fewer (as in Hoyt et al.'s (1981) protocol) muscle groups; the amount of time or number of assessments necessary to obtain reliable measures of muscle activity; and the number of positions, whether resting or moving, needed to obtain clinically useful information.

Electromyography and Headache

Research findings in the use of electromyographic measures for assessing headache pain are less encouraging than are those for assessing back pain. Results on the use of EMG as a potential aid in diagnosis are inconsistent. Some studies show higher electromyographic levels among tension and migraine headache patients as compared with nonheadache patients (e.g., Andrasik & Holroyd, 1980; Cohen Williamson, Monguillot, Hutchinson, Gottlieb, &

Waters, 1983; Cram & Steger, 1983), whereas other studies do not (e.g., Gannon, Haynes, Safranek, & Hamilton, 1981; Martin & Mathews, 1978). Also, the meaning of electromyographic levels is not clear. They usually do not correlate significantly with the experience of pain, and decreases in reported pain following electromyographic biofeedback is not necessarily associated with decreases in electromyographic activity (Epstein & Abel, 1977; Epstein, Abel, Collins, Parker, & Cinciripini, 1978; Haynes, Griffin, Mooney, & Parise, 1975; Martin & Mathews, 1978). In sum, the use of EMG as an assessment tool in headache pain has yet to be strongly supported empirically.

Electromyography and Myofacial Pain Dysfunction Syndrome

Patients with the myofacial pain dysfunction (MPD) syndrome, also called the temporomandibular joint syndrome, complain of a deep, radiating pain centered just in front of the ear. Researchers have found MPD patients to have significantly higher electromyographic levels in the masseter and temporal muscles, which are involved in chewing, than do normal subjects when performing stressful tasks (Thomas, Tiber, & Schireson, 1973; Yemm, 1969). Unfortunately, like EMG and headache, decreases in pain following treatment are not necessarily associated directly with decreases in electromyographic activity in these muscle groups (Stenn, Mothersill, & Brooke, 1979).

More positive findings have been reported with measurements of electromyographic "silent periods" in diagnosing MPD. Bessette, Bishop, and Mohl (1971) describe an assessment procedure in which a solenoid-driven plunger delivers a tap to the mandibular symphysis of MPD patients while the patient clenches his or her teeth. Electromyographic recordings of the masseter muscles are made just before and after delivery of the tap. In all individuals, the tap is associated with an immediate jaw reflex followed by an electromyographic silent period in which the muscles are inactive despite the attempt to clench. Bessette, Bishop, and Mohl (1971) found this silent period to be significantly longer for MPD patients (range 24 to 150 ms) than for normal subjects (range 20 to 30 ms). In addition, the silent period tended to increase with the severity of MPD (measured by interincisor distance), a finding replicated in another study (McCall, Uthman, & Mohl, 1978). In a group of 22 subjects (13 of whom had MPD and 9 of whom were normal) Bassette, Mohl, and DiCosimo (1974) were able to accurately classify each person as either an MPD patient or a normal subject, using a silent period of 30 ms or less to identify the normal subjects. As further evidence of the validity of the silent period, Bailey, McCall, and Ash (1977) examined 19 subjects, 10 MPD patients and 9 normal subjects, and found that 7 of the 10 MPD patients had silent periods of greater than 39 ms, while all the normal subjects had silent periods of less than 35 ms. In addition, all 7 MPD patients whose silent period was 40 ms or greater responded positively to occlusion therapy, whereas none of the 3 patients whose silent period was less than 35 ms responded. Bailey, McCall, and Ash (1977) also found the length of the silent period to correlate significantly (r=0.91) with another objective measure of the disorder: the jaw motion error.

In sum, the use of the silent period has been validated as an objective measure associated with a diagnosis of MPD, symptom severity, and positive treatment outcome.

AUTONOMIC MEASURES

Another way to clarify the nature of pain is to examine activity in the organs and systems innervated by the sympathetic portion of the autonomic nervous system. These organs and systems, which become active during the "fight or flight" response, include the heart, vascular system, pupils, and sweat glands. Researchers and clinicians interested in assessing sympathetic activity usually measure one or more of the following: heart rate, blood pressure, blood volume (as a measure of vasomotor response), skin temperature (as another measure of vasomotor response), skin resistance (believed to be associated with sweat gland activity), and pupil dilation.

Autonomic responses were measured in pain patients with a number of clinical conditions. The primary purpose was to examine the use of assessing these systems as an aide in discriminating pain patients from normal subjects or from each other (i.e., differential diagnosis), and as a means of identifying potential correlates of pain intensity. Sympathetic nervous system activity was measured using two general strategies: (a) the assessment of surface vasomotor response with thermography; and (b) the measurement of vasometer activity using photoplethysmographs, thermistors, or both. Each of these strategies will be described briefly.

Thermography

Thermography measures skin temperature, yielding an infrared (heat-sensitive) photograph of a patient's body. Because heat varies primarily as a function of blood flow, thermographs measure surface vascular activity and may be used to assess vasomotor abnormalities. In thermography, the temperature of a painful area is compared with its anatomically identical area on the opposite side of the body. If a significant (greater than 1 degree) difference in temperature is observed, then abnormal vasomotor activity is inferred. Because certain pain disorders, such as reflex sympathetic dystrophy, are associated with abnormal vasomotor activity, they can be accurately assessed using this method.

Reflex sympathetic dystrophy, also called causalgia, is a pain condition that is associated with a severe burning sensation, hyperalgesia, and temperature changes in the affected skin. In its early stages, sympathetic reflex dystrophy can be difficult to diagnose and often is mislabeled as "psychogenic". In strong support of the use of thermography, Hendler, Uematsu, and Long (1982) were able to use thermography to identify organic disorders, including reflex sympathetic dystrophy, in 43 of 224 pain patients who had initially been diagnosed as having psychogenic pain.

As further validation of thermography in the assessment of pain, LeRoy and Bruner (1982) reported that seven patients with chronic back pain also showed abnormal thermograms. Moreover, in these patients, successful treatment following induced electrical stimulation was associated with a normalizing effect on the thermographic records, suggesting that thermography may also be useful in the diagnosis and treatment outcome assessment of chronic back pain.

The thermographic measurement of pain does not involve skin contact (which can alter skin temperature and thus bias the results), is not invasive, and can be performed quickly. Also, once temperature abnormalities are identified, further thermographic assessment can be used as ipsative measures of treatment outcome. Finally, because of its ability to identify abnormalities in some pain disorders, especially in their early stages of development, thermography is an excellent tool for the diagnosis and screening of some chronic pain states.

Blood Flow or Blood Volume

The most common methods of measuring vasomotor activity involve a photoplethysmograph (Kallman & Feuerstein, 1977), a thermistor, or both. The photoplethysmograph measures the amount of light shining through or reflecting from tissue. The more blood in the tissue, the less light is reflected. The thermistor converts skin temperature to an electrical signal that can be amplified and displayed. Most commonly, the photoplethysmograph is used to assess vasomotor responding in cranial arteries, while the thermistor is used to measure vasomotor activity in peripheral arteries (usually in a finger or hand).

Research supports the conclusion that migraine headaches are associated with abnormal responding in the cranial arteries (cf. Bakal, 1975). Migraine headaches generally are associated with vasoconstriction in the cranial arteries several hours before the headache and with vasodilation during the experience of headache pain. Changes in vasomotor activity may actually be preceded by vasodilation 3 days before the migraine attack (Feuerstein, Bortolussi, Houle, & Labbé, 1983).

If migraine headache sufferers indeed demonstrate abnormal cranial vasomotor responding, they possibly also evidence a generalized disorder of the vascular system. Measuring vasomotor responding in the arteries other than those in the head, therefore, may be important in the assessment of migraine. Unfortunately, evidence is contradictory regarding abnormalities in the hand vasculature of migraine sufferers. Some studies show that migraine sufferers demonstrate abnormal hand vasomotor responding (e.g., Appenzeller, 1969; Appenzeller, Davison, & Marshall, 1963; Downey & Frewin, 1972; Elliot, Frewin, & Downey, 1974), and some have been unable to detect differences between migraine sufferers and normal subjects (e.g., French, Lassers, & Desai, 1967; Hockaday, Macmillan, & Whitty, 1967).

Overall, measures of cranial vasomotor responding have demonstrated more potential as an aid in the assessment of migraine headache than has measurement of hand vasomotor responding. However, clear clinical applications of cranial blood volume measures have yet to be developed.

MULTIPLE PHYSIOLOGICAL MEASUREMENT

The final method of assessment involves multiple physiologic measures. For example, Cohen et al. (1983) measured heart rate, skin potential, cephalic vasomotor responding, finger skin temperature, and frontalis electromyographic activity among four groups of headache sufferers (muscle contraction, common migraine, classic migraine, and mixed) and a group of normal subjects in response to relaxation and stress. The important finding of this well-designed study is that the different experimental groups demonstrated different patterns of responding, especially under stress. Entering the physiological measures into a discriminant function to predict the type of headache, they were able to correctly classify 67% of the patients (only 25% of the patients would be expected to be correctly classified by chance alone). Classification using the physiological measures was better than the interrater reliability based on the diagnosis by each patient's personal physician.

Although the results of the Cohen et al. (1983) study are promising, such findings are rare in the literature. Andrasik, Blanchard, Arena, Saunders, and Barron (1982) measured frontalis and forearm EMG, temporal artery blood flow, hand surface temperature, heart rate, and skin resistance among migraine, tension, mixed, and control subjects during rest, self-control (told to relax their body, warm their hands, and relax their forehead), and stress conditions. They found no consistent patterns of responding among the headache patients and were only able to correctly classify 41% of the subjects using the physiological measures in a discriminant function analysis.

Bakal and Kaganov (1977) measured frontalis EMG, neck EMG, and pulse velocities from the right and left temporal arteries in migraine and headache sufferers during both headache and headache-free periods, and obtained the same measures on two occasions from nonheadache subjects. Measurements were made during relaxation and during the random presentation of a nonaversive white noise. Migraine sufferers had a higher level of frontalis EMG during both the headache and headache-free conditions, whereas the electromyographic measures were not different among the tension headache and control subjects. They also found pulse velocity in the left temporal artery to decrease in response to the white noise in both headache subjects relative to control subjects. These findings differ from those of Cohen et al. (1983) who found that vasomotor responding did not play a larger role than other physiological measures in differentiating headache from nonheadache subjects, and that EMG did not reliably differentiate muscle contraction headache sufferers from migraine sufferers.

In a third study, Gannon, Haynes, Safranek, and Hamilton (1981) measured frontal EMG, forearm EMG, earlobe blood volume, and heart rate in migraine patients, tension headache patients, and control subjects during rest, stress, and poststress adaptation. They found no differences between the groups on the electromyographic measures. However, they did find that the migraine sufferers tended to demonstrate greater vasoconstriction during the adaptation period than did the nonheadache control subjects, replicating the findings of Bakal and Kaganov (1977) but not those of Cohen et al. (1983).

Cohen and colleagues, in an attempt to explain their overall positive findings compared with the generally negative findings in other studies, point out three important differences between their study and those of others: (a) they selected more extreme cases of headache and nonheadache patients; (b) they had a longer relaxation phase; and (c) they had a longer and more intense stressful phase.

In sum, although multiple measures of physiological responding may have some clinical as well as theoretical use in the assessment of headache pain, additional well-controlled studies are needed to establish the usefulness of this approach.

SUMMARY

In this chapter, several of the most commonly used biophysical measures of clinical pain are discussed and critiqued. Some of the methods show promise as indices of key physiological correlates of pain. In particular, the use of thermography in diagnosing reflex sympathetic dystrophy and back pain and the use of electromyographic silent periods in diagnosing myofacial pain disorder have been supported. Also, both percutaneous neurography and biochemical measures of endorphin activity have been helpful in understanding specific pain states and their physiological correlates, supporting the continued development of these methods for use by the clinician.

Chapter 6
Behavioral Observation Methods

When patients demonstrate the intensity of their pain behaviorally, such as by complaints and grimacing, and when they engage in specific actions to cope with it (such as taking medications and resting), they reveal the complex, multilayered nature of their suffering, and challenge assessors to find methods capable of reliably quantifying their experience.

Pain-related behaviors may reflect not only the extent of a patient's pain, but may also serve to impede recovery from chronic pain syndromes. Pain behavior is often followed by social reinforcement (e.g., solicitous statements and extra tender loving care) or narcotic medications, which some persons find highly rewarding. Patients may likewise perceive that financial compensation, in the form of disability payments, depends on their continued experience and expression of pain. Because it is well known that behaviors followed by positive or rewarding events tend to increase in frequency, certain pain responses can tend to increase even when perceived pain intensity is decreasing (cf. Fordyce, 1976). Patients who frequently enact pain-related behaviors typically experience longer periods of disability and decreased opportunities for a pain-free life.

This chapter begins with an introduction to issues important in the assessment of discrete, ongoing behavior. Specific pain behaviors amenable to observational assessment are then introduced, and various methods for counting, recording, and coding such behaviors are discussed and critiqued.

ISSUES IN BEHAVIORAL OBSERVATION

Any assessment procedure, if it is to provide meaningful information, must be both reliable and valid. First, the same observational procedure used by different judges or, by the same person at different times, should yield essentially the same results, that is, it should be reliable. Second, an assessment procedure should measure what it professes to, that is, it should be valid. This is usually determined by comparing an observer's record with a distinct, independently measured (criterion) index of the same behavior.

There are many potential threats to the reliability and validity of observational procedures (cf. Jeffrey, 1974; Nelson, 1977; Wildman & Erickson, 1977). To reduce the potential effects of these threats in the assessment of pain behavior, the following seven guidelines should be observed as closely as possible.

1. Select clearly defined target behaviors. Behaviors that are vaguely defined (e.g., looking uncomfortable) are much more difficult to code reliably than are actions specifically defined (e.g., rubbing neck). The more vaguely defined the behavior, the less likely two observers will agree on its occurrence. Behaviors to be coded should be defined as observable events, be clear (readable and unambiguous), and be complete and indicate the boundaries of inclusion and exclusion (Hawkins & Dobes, 1977).

2. Provide training. Persons are not naturally accurate and reliable observers of ongoing behavior. Observers need to be trained and allowed to practice observational and recording procedures. Training should continue until an observer reaches a minimum level of reliability, usually judged as an accuracy rate of 80%.

   Several procedures can make training more effective. First, immediate accuracy feedback should be provided to trainees so they will quickly appreciate when they are and are not recording correctly (Mahoney & Thoresen, 1974). Second, observers should have the opportunity to practice under conditions that closely resemble the settings in which actual observations will take place (Wildman & Erickson, 1977). Third, because observer expectations can affect what is seen, observers should not be led to expect specific behaviors from pain patients. Fourth, to control for observer drift, that is, the tendency of observers to alter, in idiosyncratic ways, how they observe and/or record behavior over time — retraining of observers (against a standard or criterion level) should occur at regular intervals, at least every few weeks. Finally, because reliability increases when observers are aware that their accuracy is being monitored, it is important that observer accuracy be verified regularly (cf. Nelson, 1977). Regular accuracy checks may also be used to gauge the necessity of retraining.

3. Control for patient reactivity. Reactivity refers to the tendency of people's behavior to change when they know they are being observed. To control for patient reactivity, observers should be instructed to be as unobtrusive as possible and to refrain from social contact (e.g., conversation and eye contact) with the pain patient during observation periods.

4. Limit the work load of the observers. Research indicates that observers can code pain behaviors more reliably when there are fewer behaviors to observe and code (e.g., 7) than when there are many behaviors to keep track of (e.g., 16) (Follick, Ahern, & Aberger, 1985).

5. Sample representative behaviors. If an adequate sample of the pain patient's natural lifespace has not been observed, there is an increased likelihood that the behaviors being observed will not adequately represent the patient's usual or typical modes of response. Pain patients can have bad days, and pain can vary systematically throughout the day (Folkard, Glynn, & Lloyd, 1976). To assess a single patient's pain behavior, then, multiple assessments of behavior should be made at different times of the day and on different days.

6. Record the behavior as soon as possible after observing it. The longer the time between the observing and recording of behavior, the less reliable the coding of that behavior may become.

7. Keep the observation procedure simple and clear (particularly for self-observation). Accurate observation can be a difficult and sometimes tedious task. To increase compliance and reliability, the observation procedures should be as straightforward as possible. Rather than asking patients to record their own behavior every half hour for many weeks, for example, we recommend that patients be asked to record their pain levels and behavior at four convenient times during the day (such as just after awakening, before lunch, before dinner, and before going to sleep at night). In addition, we recommend that behavior recorders, especially in the case of self-observation, be supplied with all the necessary materials for observing and coding such as pens and data sheets (Fordyce, 1976).

These seven guidelines should be considered necessary, but not sufficient, for the development of valid and reliable behavioral observation procedures.

A LIST OF PAIN BEHAVIORS

Many different behaviors may be observed in the pain patient. A partial list of these is presented in Table 6.1. We have classified them into three major types: (a) pain communication behaviors; (b) pain-coping behaviors; and (c) lifestyle pain behaviors. Pain communication behaviors, such as guarding, grimacing, and asking for medications, provide a measure of pain intensity as well as a measure of pain communication style. The assessment of pain-coping behaviors, such as relaxation, medication use, and exercise, can provide an indirect measure of pain intensity as well as an index of the general coping style of the patient (e.g., active versus passive). Finally, measures of lifestyle pain behaviors, such as time spent working, mobility and strength, and sleeping habits, allow for a relational assessment of how the pain patient is currently being affected by the pain condition and can be used to index the overall quality of life. The three categories listed should not be considered necessarily distinct, because a single behavior can sometimes fit into more than one category. For

Table 6.1. List of Behaviors Associated with Chronic Pain

Pain Communication Behaviors	Pain-Coping Behaviors	Pain Lifestyle Behaviors
Guarding	Biofeedback/relaxation	Work–nonwork
Grimacing	Medication use	Mobility–immobility
Rubbing	Exercise/yoga	Strength
Sighing	Help seeking	Social activities
Partial movement	Rest/inactivity	Sexual activities
Limitation statements	Counterstimulation	Recreation/hobbies
Sounds	Attention diversion	Sleep
Position shifting	Rubbing	Time at home
Bracing	Bracing	Uptime/downtime
Asking for medications	Guarding	Position
	Position shifting	Exercise tolerance
		Household chores

example, rubbing may be considered both a pain communication and a pain-coping behavior.

BEHAVIORAL OBSERVATION METHODS

Several procedures have been developed to quantify the kinds of behaviors listed in Table 6.1. These include the use of structured pain behavior observations, hospital and in vivo behavior observations, self-monitoring, measures of medication intake, electromechanical assessment, and physical performance measures.

Structured Pain Behavior Observation

A structured pain behavior observational procedure may be used to assess both verbal and nonverbal pain communication behaviors. The procedure usually involves requesting that the patient engage in a standard set of tasks and then respond to a standard set of questions. Usually, patients are videotaped and their elicited behaviors and comments are later coded by trained observers. Before the assessment can begin, the clinician selects the target behaviors to be observed and the tasks for the patient to perform, chooses data recording procedures, and trains the observers.

Selection of Target Behaviors

There is yet insufficient research to support the exclusive use of any specific subset of pain communication behaviors. However, some preliminary research indicates that certain behaviors can be reliably measured and can discriminate pain from nonpain patients. These are the five pain behaviors employed in the work of Keefe and his colleagues (cf. Keefe & Block, 1982) including guarding, bracing, rubbing, grimacing, and sighing. Other behaviors that have demonstrated adequate psychometric properties include partial movement, limitation statements, sounds, and position shifts (Follick, Ahern, & Aberger, 1985). Until research supports the use of other specific target behaviors, we recommend that Keefe's five behaviors be used because, to date, these behaviors have been the most extensively studied and supported.

Choosing the Assessment Procedures

To insure that the structure of the observation procedures remains the same across pain patients, the tasks and questions asked of the patients should be identical. The procedures used by Keefe and Block (1982), Cinciripini and Floreen (1983), and Follick, Ahern, and Aberger (1985) provide examples that the clinician may emulate in developing his or her own procedure. Keefe and Block (1982) instruct patients to sit for two periods of time (1 and 2 minutes), stand for two periods (1 and 2 minutes), walk for two periods (two 1-minute periods), and recline for two periods (two 1-minute periods), resulting in an assessment session that lasts 10 minutes. An order of tasks is chosen so that patients are not required to perform the same task for two consecutive periods.

Cinciripini and Floreen (1983) interview their patients for 20 minutes and ask four questions, to which the patients are allowed 3 minutes to respond and are prompted if they pause for more than 20 seconds. The four questions are:

1. Tell me about your pain. Describe it in detail — what makes it better or worse. What brings it on. When it started — things like that.
2. Describe the things you like to do, like leisure activity, hobbies, social gatherings, and sports, and how often you do them.
3. Tell me about your family (wife or husband). How do they respond to your pain, what do they do, and how do they know you are hurting? How has the pain affected you relationship?
4. Tell me about your personality. What are your strengths, what things do you like about yourself, and what are your resources?

Following the questions, the patients are asked to rise from their chair, walk around the room, pick up an ashtray from the floor, and pick up and carry a chair several feet.

Follick, Ahern, and Aberger (1985) require patients to perform a series of behaviors, including sitting, standing, walking, bending, and various exercises, and to respond to two questions. The two questions they ask are: "Describe your average day" and "What are your hobbies and interests, and how often do you engage in them?"

In each of the foregoing procedures, patients are observed for at least 5 minutes at a time. Although procedures of less duration have been used in some research, we believe that a minimum of at least 5 minutes is necessary to provide an adequate sampling of behavior.

If the clinician decides to include questions as part of the interview, it should be noted that the kind of question asked may influence the frequency of pain behaviors observed. Specifically, pain-neutral subjects (such as questions about the patients' personality or about things they like to do) appear to elicit few pain communication behaviors, whereas pain-related questions (such as asking patients to describe their pain and how others respond to it) appear to elicit relatively higher frequencies of overt pain behavior (Cinciripini & Floreen, 1983). Ideally, once the procedures (target behaviors, tasks, and questions) have been selected, all interviews would be videotaped. Videotaping permits the accumulation of materials for use in observer training and also provides a permanent record of the patient's behavior, which can help verify observer reliability, demonstrate behavior changes over time (e.g., before to after treatment), and code the behaviors, should trained observers not be available during the actual interview. However, videotaping may not always be practical or affordable. Also, research indicates that observers can reliably code pain behaviors in vivo, making videotaping unnecessary (Keefe, Wilkins, & Cook, 1984). However, regular retraining of observers as well as regular checks on reliability should occur regardless of whether raters will be observing tapes or live behaviors.

We recommend the observation procedure employed by Keefe and his colleagues (cf. Keefe & Block, 1982). This method involves alternating between observing (for 20 seconds) and coding (for 10 seconds). For a 10-minute interview, 20 blocks of behavior are observed, and the occurrence or nonoccurrence of target behaviors are indicated on a coding sheet.

Training the Observers

Training may be accomplished by having trainees carefully study a manual that outlines the observation procedures and provides clear definitions of the behaviors to be recorded. Training tapes, which have been previously coded, can be used by the trainee until he or she consistently reaches an adequate level of agreement, usually 80% with the expert or criterion scoring. If training tapes are not available, two trainees can observe the same patients until they reach an adequate agreement with each other. Once training is completed, the observation of pain communication behaviors can begin. Remember to provide ongoing training to reduce the possibility of observer drift and also remember to perform periodic observer reliability checks.

Hospital Ward and In Vivo Observation

The major criticism of structured pain behavior observation procedures is that patient activity is observed in a highly controlled environment. Although control can provide greater reliability of measurement, the 5-, 10-, or even 20-minute observation period may well represent only a small slice of the patient's total life. In addition, the patient is observed while performing tasks he or she has been asked to perform, rather than during the course of an ordinary day. Therefore, the behaviors observed may not represent the usual pain behaviors of the patient. Hospital and in vivo observational procedures were developed to assess pain behavior in a somewhat more naturalistic setting, that is, one relatively unconstrained by experimental instruction, but nonetheless subject to environmental (setting-specific) constraints.

Choosing the Target Behaviors and Assessment Procedures

Nearly all of the behaviors listed in Table 6.1 may be assessed by in vivo observational procedures. The clinician must simply choose those behaviors deemed most important and remember to limit the choice enough so that the observers are not overwhelmed by their duties. Behaviors most often assessed by hospital-based in vivo observations include medication use, uptime and downtime, and time spent in various positions, such as sitting and standing. These behaviors provide indicators of how the patient's pain is affecting his or her hospital adaptation, and they may be measured by self-monitoring procedures as well (see below). One advantage of employing trained observers to assess pain behaviors is that the data so obtained can be used to cross-check the reliability of patient self-observations. Observers may also tend to increase the reliability of the self-monitoring assessments. (Recall that persons tend to be more accurate when they believe that another person is observing and recording the same behaviors.)

For recording behaviors, such as position and activity, that can occur any time throughout the day, a sampling time frame should be selected that captures the "window of opportunity" for representative observation. On an inpatient ward, for example, a staff person may be assigned to observe the patient on every shift and at selected times throughout the shift, perhaps for 5 minutes of each half hour (cf. Cinciripini & Floreen, 1982). Behaviors that occur infrequently or at specific times (e.g., the ingestion of medications or use of biofeedback) should be precisely scheduled for observation and recorded as they occur.

Self-Monitoring of Pain Behavior: The Pain Diary

Self-monitoring of pain behavior is the most widely used behavior observation method, probably because the procedure is: (a) very inexpensive (no observers need be hired), (b) easy to administer (the patient does much of the work), and (c) provides the only possible way to sample the entire behavioral repertoire of the patient — the patient is always there when he or she emits a pain behavior. Two kinds of pain diaries have been employed, (a) those that assess specific pain behavior, and (b) those that provide for functional assessment.

Specific Pain Behavior Diary

Fordyce and his colleagues were perhaps the first to use the pain diary as an assessment tool (cf. Fordyce, Fowler, Lehmann, DeLateur, Sand, & Trieschmann, 1973). Fordyce and his associates ask patients to record the time spent in one of three positions: reclining, standing/walking, or sitting, during their waking hours. Also, on a daily activity sheet, patients are asked to record the occurrence or nonoccurrence of a number of activities, including visiting (from or to relatives or others), outside-home trips, and inside-home activities.

A similar diary requires patients to keep a record of their position, time spent alone or with others, time at home, medication use, pain-coping behaviors, and subjective pain level (Follick, Ahern, & Laser-Wolston, 1984). The diary is organized into one-hour time blocks, allowing patients to indicate their behavior throughout the day. At three times during the day, that is, 12 noon, 5 pm, and before retiring, patients are asked to recall the physical position in which they spent most of their time during each one-hour period, to list and describe the activity in which they spent most of the time block, to indicate how they spent their time (e.g., at home and alone), to list any medications taken, and to indicate any pain-coping activities performed. An example of a pain diary that incorporates some of the best features of other diaries is presented in Figure 6.1.

We ask our patients to report their activities four times a day. Although it may seem unnecessary to ask the patient to record position, medication use, and activities during the period between retiring and arising, many pain patients do not necessarily spend this time sleeping. During that time, medications can be taken, the patient may be reclining but still awake, or the patient may get out of bed. If we wait until noon to ask the patient to record what he or she did during the night as well as in the time between waking and noon, we may lose some of the details of behavior during the night. In addition, it is useful to have measures of pain intensity first thing in the morning, so as to assess its diurnal variations.

Day: _____

Midnight	Pain	Pos. code	Med. code	Act./ Loc. code
12–1				
1–2				
2–3				
3–4				
4–5				
AM 5–6				
6–7				
7–8				
8–9				
9–10				
10–11				
11–12				
Noon–1				
1–2				
2–3				
3–4				
4–5				
PM 5–6				
6–7				
7–8				
8–9				
9–10				
10–11				
11–12				

Date: _____

Instructions: At four times during the day (when you awaken, before lunch, before dinner, and before you go to sleep) record your perceived pain intensity on a 0 ("no pain") to 100 ("pain as bad as it could be") scale. Then think about what you did since the last time you made a diary entry and indicate: (1) the position you spent the most time in during each hour block; (2) the activity you performed and where you were during each hour block; and (3) the kind and dose of any medications you took for pain relief. Use the codes below to write in your diary.

Position codes:
  1 = Sitting.
  2 = Reclining/awake.
  3 = Reclining/asleep.
  4 = Walking/standing.

Medication codes:
  1 = Non-prescription analgesic:
    (_____)
  2 = Prescription analgesic:
    (_____)
  3 = Prescription analgesic:
    (_____)
  4 = Other pain medication:
    (_____)
  5 = Other pain medication:
    (_____)

Activity/location codes:
  1 = Sleeping.
  2 = Resting alone.
  3 = Resting with others.
  4 = Socializing with friends.
  5 = Socializing with family.
  6 = Working at a paying job.
  7 = Performing household chores.
  8 = Doing a hobby.
  9 = Watching TV.
  A = Inside/around my home.
  B = Away from my home.

FIGURE 6.1. Pain diary.

Functional Assessment Diary

Functional assessment diaries can be used to understand events that may precipitate a pain episode and to assess the degree to which reinforcers may follow pain reactions. Such diaries include space to record events that occur just before and just after a pain display. An example of a functional assessment diary is presented in Figure 6.2.

Day: _____ Date: _____

Time: _____ Pain intensity level (0–100): _____

What primary activity have you been performing during the last hour? _____
_____

What person or persons have you been with during the last hour? _____
_____

In what locale were you mostly during the past hour? _____
_____

How would you rate your mood during the past hour (circle)?

Sad 0 1 2 3 4 5 6 7 8 9 10 Happy

What have you been thinking during the past hour? _____
_____

What are you doing *now*? _____

Who is with you *now*? _____

To what degree are the people with whom you are now interacting treating you with care and concern (giving you enough Tender Loving Care)?

Very little 0 1 2 3 4 5 6 7 8 9 10 Very much

What are the people you are with (if anyone) specifically doing with you or for you?
_____
_____

If you are in pain, are you doing anything to relieve it?

If yes, what are you doing? _____
_____

Wait ½ to 1 hour.

Time: _____ Pain intensity level (0–100): _____
_____

FIGURE 6.2. Functional assessment diary.

The diary may be filled out as often as the patient and clinician wish. The more diaries completed, the better the patient/clinician team will be able to assess the events that are associated with pain onset and that consistently follow (reinforce or punish) the response. To provide an adequate sample, we recommend that patients complete the diary at different times, both when in pain and when not in pain. Ideally, the patient should complete the diary at random times to capture both pain and nonpain episodes. Once potential pain-related antecedents and consequences are identified, the clinician and the patient may use this information to develop a treatment plan. Although not all the events associated with increases in pain should be avoided (i.e., some exercise may produce pain in the short run but reduce it in the long run) or all reinforcers removed (the availability of reinforcers is an important aspect of a successful relationship), the data from a functional assessment diary may suggest avenues of change. For example, if the patient knows that certain, perhaps necessary, activities will bring on pain, he or she may be better able to prepare for the ensuing pain after the performance of those activities. In addition, reinforcers for pain or pain behaviors may be systematically transformed into reinforcers for decreases in pain and pain behavior (cf. Fordyce, 1976).

Medication Use and Misuse

Drug misuse is frequent among pain patients and is often employed as a behavioral index of pain treatment effectiveness or lack thereof.

Choosing the Assessment Procedures

Regardless of who observes and records drug use behavior, whether it be the patient, hospital staff, or spouse, a major decision in the measurement of drug taking concerns data coding. Many different classes and potencies of drugs are available to reduce pain, making it difficult to compare medication use between patients or within the same patient at different times. Five methods have been used to enhance the comparability of drug use information: pill counts, use and nonuse of categorized drugs, ratings, unit potency coding, and medication index scoring. We currently employ a sixth method that combines the strengths of some of the methods already in use.

1. Pill counts: The pill count procedure involves the summing of the number of pills ingested over a specified period such as a day or a week. We do not recommend this procedure, despite its simplicity, because information on specific doses and the kinds of drugs used can readily be lost.
2. Use or nonuse of categorized drugs: A second method involves coding the

use and nonuse of each of a number of distinct classes of drugs. Classes of drugs can include narcotics, nonnarcotic analgesics, muscle relaxants, mild tranquilizers, antidepressants, and antianxiety agents. This method is appropriate for obtaining a general sense of the pattern of drug use. A person who begins treatment with narcotics and completes treatment taking only nonprescription analgesics, or no drugs at all, might well be considered a treatment success. The major problem with this method is that another patient may be taking few narcotics at the beginning of treatment (e.g., one per week) and many nonnarcotic analgesics after treatment (e.g., 10 per day). Under these circumstances, labeling the treatment outcome *successful* may be questioned.

3. Ratings: Several clinicians and researchers have developed rating scales for assessing drug use. One system assigns patients a 1 for taking the maximum prescribed dose of a prescription pain medication, such as opiate derivatives, synthetic opiates, hypnotics, sedatives, and tranquilizers. Those taking 50% or less of the maximum prescribed dose are given a rating of 2. A rating of 3 is applied to patients taking a prescribed pain medication occasionally and to those taking up to 100% of the maximum dose of a nonprescription analgesic (such as aspirin), and a rating of 4 is assigned to patients taking no prescription medications and those using only an occasional nonprescription analgesic (Gottlieb, Strite, Koller, Madorsky, Hockersmith, Kleeman, & Wagner, 1977). The strength of this method is that it allows for comparisons among patients taking different pain medications at different doses. Unfortunately, by combining classes of drugs, a patient who is experiencing pain and taking 100% of the maximum dose of a nonprescription analgesic could be rated as doing better than a patient who feels no pain but who is taking a hypnotic to assist him or her in going to sleep. The rating method is therefore probably best used for comparing drug use among groups of patients.

4. Unit potency values: Another system assesses drug use with respect to its potential analgesic effects, using morphine as the standard (cf. Fordyce et al., 1973). With this approach, the average effective dose of a medication is divided into the average effective dose of morphine (10 mg every 4 hours) to create a potency value for each pain medication. For example, the potency value for morphine is 1, whereas the potency value for codeine, which has an average effective dose of 60 mg every 4 hours, is one-sixth or 0.17. The potency values computed for each drug may then be multiplied by the dose(s) of the drug(s) currently being taken daily by a pain patient, and then summed to create the unit potency dose for that patient. This method is more complicated than those described thus far and requires highly accurate recordings of drug use by the patient. However, the method is also useful in gauging the analgesic levels being experienced by patients.

5. Medication index: The medication index is an attempt to provide a sensitive

but simple method of scoring overall drug use (Blanchard & Andrasik, 1985). Pain medications are first scored according to their general potency. Aspirin-like analgesics and antiinflammatory medications are given a score of 1, mild narcotic analgesics a score of 2, antianxiety and antidepressants a score of 3, codeine and codeine-like narcotic analgesics a score of 4, demerol (meperidine) 5, Dilaudid (Hydromorphone) and morphine or Nuvaine a score of 7.

To compute a patient's medication index, the dosage of each pain medication is multiplied by the score for that medication and the total summed. For example, a patient who takes four aspirin tablets and 1 antianxiety tablet a day would have a daily medication index of 7.

The major problem with the medication index method is that a single dose of one drug may be twice as strong as a dose of another drug in the same category. For example, a patient taking three Tylenol IIIs would have the same medication index (12) as would a patient taking three Tylenol IVs, even though the latter patient is ingesting twice as much codeine. Therefore, the scores assigned the various medications are somewhat arbitrary. Why do antianxiety medications have a score three times that of aspirin and half that of Dilaudid?

6. Drug measure: Because of our dissatisfaction with current measures of drug use, we have developed an additional coding method which we have found to be helpful. It is essentially a simplified version of the unit potency approach just described. First, the method involves categorizing medications into one of six kinds of drugs taken by pain patients: (a) nonnarcotic analgesics and antiinflammatory drugs; (b) narcotic analgesics; (c) antidepressants; (d) antianxiety drugs; (e) hypnotics (sleeping pills); and (f) muscle relaxants/antispasm drugs. We then consult a reference, usually the *Physician's Desk Reference*, about the usual total daily allowable dose for the drug. This is defined as the usual daily maintenance dose listed for the drug. If a range of the usual daily dose is given rather than a single dose, the upper end of the range becomes the daily allowable dose for that drug. If no range is given, then the listed maximum recommended dose is used. The usual allowable daily doses of many common drugs given to pain patients are presented in Table 6.2.

Patients are asked to carefully record the daily dose of each drug they are taking. The actual daily dose of each drug being taken is divided by the daily allowable dose of that drug and multiplied by 100. This quantity, which we call the drug measure, can be thought of as a percentage of the maximum daily allowable dose for each drug. If it is greater than 100, then the patient is taking more than is usually recommended. We prefer to sum the drug measures of each drug taken within drug categories and not between them. This allows separate calculation of drug use across the distinct categories of medication. However, it certainly would be possible to average the drug

Table 6.2. Allowable Daily Doses for Common Drugs Given to Pain Patients

Drug Name	Products that Include the Drug	Allowable Daily Dose (mg)
Nonnarcotic Analgesics and Antiinflammatory Drugs		
Acetaminophen	Tylenol, Excedrin	4,000
Acetylsalicylic acid (ASA)	Anacin, Aspirin, Bufferin, Excedrin, etc.	4,000
Diflunisal	Dolobid	1,500
Ibuprofen	Advil, Motrin, Nuprin	3,200
Indomethacin	Indocin	200
Naproxen	Anaprox, Naprosyn	1,375
Piroxicam	Feldene	20
Sulindac	Clinoril	400
Tolmetin sodium	Tolectin	1,800
Narcotic Analgesics		
Codeine phosphate	Empirin w/Codeine, Soma Compound w/Codeine, Tylenol III, IV	360
Hydrocodone bitartrate	Vicodin	40
Hydromorphone HCl	Dilaudid (IM)	12
Meperidine HCl	Demerol (IM)	900
Morphine sulfate	Duramorph (IV)	
Oxycodone HCl	Percocet, Percodan, Tylox	20
Oxymorphone HCl	Numorphan	9
Propoxyphene HCl	Darvon	390
Propoxyphene napsylate	Darvocet-N, Darvon-N	600
Muscle Relaxants/Antispasm Medications		
Baclofen	Lioresal	80
Butalbital	Fiorinal	300
Carisoprodol	Soma, Soma Compound	1,600
Chlorzoxazone	Parafon forte	2,000
Cyclobenzaprine HCl	Flexeril	40
Diazepam	Valium	40
Metaxalone	Skelaxin	3,200
Methocarbamol	Robaxin, Robaxisal	4,000
Antidepressants		
Amitriptyline HCl	Elavil, Endep, Etrafron, Limbitrol, Triavil	150
Amoxapine	Asendin	300
Desipramine HCl	Norpramin, Pertofrane	200
Doxepin HCl	Adapin, Sinequan	150
Imipramine HCl	Tofranil	150
Isocarboxazid	Marplan	20
Maprotiline HCl	Ludiomil	150
Nortriptyline HCl	Aventyl, Pamelor	150
Phenelzine sulfate	Nardil	15
Protriptyline HCl	Vivactil	40

Tranylcypromine sulfate	Parnate	20
Trazodone HCl	Desyrel	400
Trimipramine maleate	Surmontil	150

Antianxiety Medications

Alprazolam	Xanax	4
Chlordiazepoxide	Libritabs, Limbitrol	40
Chlordiazepoxide HCl	Librium	40
Clorazepate dipotassium	Tranxene	30
Diazepam	Valium	40
Doxepin HCl	Adapin, Sinequan	150
Halazepam	Paxipam	160
Hydroxyzine HCl	Atarax, Durrax	400
Hydroxyzine pamoate	Vistaril	400
Lorazepam	Ativan	6
Meprobamate	Equagesic, Equanil, Meprospan, Miltown	1,600
Oxazepam	Serax	120
Prazepam	Centrax	30

Hypnotics (sleeping medications)

Chloral hydrate	Noctec	1,000
Ethchlorvynol	Placidyl	500
Ethinamate	Valmid	1,000
Flurazepam HCl	Dalmane	30
Secobarbital sodium	Seconal	100
Temazepam	Restoril	30
Triazolam	Halcion	0.5

Note. The allowable daily dose listed is the maximum dose recommended by the drug's listing in the Physician's Drug Reference and does not necessarily represent the dose that should be administered on one occasion. This table should be used only to calculate drug measures for pain patients. Never should the table be used as a guide for prescribing medications.

measures across some or all of the categories, if a more general measure of drug use were desired.

To illustrate the method, let us assume that a patient is taking 4 Soma Compound (carisprodol and aspirin) with codeine tablets and 150 mg of Sinequan (Doxepin) a day. This means that the patient is ingesting 800 mg of carisoprodol (muscle relaxant), 1,300 mg of aspirin (nonnarcotic analgesic), 64 mg of codeine phosphate (narcotic analgesic), and 150 mg of Doxepin (antidepressant) daily. By dividing the dose being taken by the daily allowable dose of each of these drugs and multiplying by 100, we calculate drug measures of 50% for muscle relaxants ($800 \div 1,600 \times 100$), 33% for nonnarcotic analgesics ($1,300 \div 4,000 \times 100$), 18% for narcotic analgesics ($64 \div 360 \times 100$), and 100% for antidepressants ($150 \div 150 \times 100$). We are now in a position to compare this patient's medication use within specific drug categories with his or her use at different times or with the use of other patients.

It should be remembered that patients may tend to underestimate medication use, especially if they perceive disapproval for using drugs to control pain. Therefore, it is wise to corroborate patients' self-report with biochemical assays or reports from informants, or both.

Electromechanical Devices

Although mechanical devices may be used to measure only a small subset of the behaviors listed in Table 6.1, that subset is measured extremely well, arguing for use of the devices whenever practical. The four kinds of pain behavior that have been assessed with the assistance of mechanical devices are activity level, position, uptime, and gait patterns.

Activity Level

A pedometer gauges the distance traversed by the person wearing it, usually attached to his or her belt. Although pedometers have not yet been widely employed to measure activity levels in pain patients, we recommend their use because of their availability and low cost (Cinciripini & Floreen, 1982). These instruments may be calibrated to match the stride of an individual patient, making possible between-patient comparisons in activity levels. Unfortunately, patients who shake the pedometer can cause it to measure more walking than actually took place. We therefore recommend that additional indices of activity level be employed whenever possible.

Position

A device has been developed that employs a miniature electronic timer wired to a tilt switch mounted on the outer thigh of a pain patient (Sanders, 1980). The timer starts whenever the leg is horizontal, which occurs when the patient sits or lies down and stops when the leg is vertical, which occurs when the patient is standing or walking. Thus, the device assesses the total time spent lying down and sitting (the time observed on the timer) or standing and walking (the time since the timer was reset minus that observed on the timer). The device has demonstrated both its reliability and its validity as a measure of position.

Uptime and Downtime

Two devices have been used to measure uptime and downtime. The first involves equipping a patient's bed with a microswitch that starts a clock whenever the patient sits or lies down upon it (Cairns, Thomas, Mooney, &

Pace, 1976). Because the clock is readily visible, the patient is able to see exactly how much time he or she has spent in or on the bed during the course of a day. This method is excellent for encouraging patients to stay out of bed, although it does not assess the amount of time spent in any particular position.

A second device employs a position switch mounted on the patient's waist, so that the timer runs only when the patient is lying down (Follick, Ahern, Laser-Wolston, Adams, & Molloy, 1985). This device measures the time spent lying down regardless of where the patient elects to do so. Follick et al. (1985) found that the device is both reliable and valid as an index of uptime and downtime.

Gait

A fourth electromechanical device, the Krusen Dual Force Monitor, uses pressure-sensitive insoles to record the weight on each foot over time (Keefe & Hill, 1985). The insoles are placed in the patient's shoes and the patient is asked to walk a specified distance. Three gait measures, closely associated with one another, may be obtained from the record of walking produced by the device: (a) swing time: the elapsed time between the toe leaving the ground and the heel of the same foot touching the ground; (b) single limb support time: the time the foot is *flat* against the ground; (c) stance time: the time the foot is touching the ground. In addition, the weight pattern record may be helpful in measuring: (d) step length: the distance between the heels of the right and left feet while walking; (e) stride length: the distance between two heel strikes of a particular foot. Velocity may also be assessed by dividing the total distance walked by the time taken to walk that distance.

Keefe and Hill (1985) found discriminative validity for measures of velocity, stride length, and step length, in that these measures were significantly different in chronic low back pain patients, compared with nonpain patients. Chronic pain patients tend to walk more slowly and have shorter step and stride lengths. In addition, much similarity was found among measures of swing time, single limb support time, and stance time between the left and right feet in normal subjects, whereas a discrepancy was found between the left and right feet in chronic low back pain patients. Pain patients displayed greater asymmetry, that is, they limped more. The pressure-sensitive insoles may prove to be excellent in assessing outcome for treatments designed to affect pain behavior and gait.

PHYSICAL PERFORMANCE

Clinicians and researchers have sought to measure two basic categories of physical performance: exercise tolerance and mobility. Most often, the measurement of these behaviors is carried out by trained physical therapists.

Exercise Tolerance

To be measurable, exercise must be reduced to a movement cycle that can be counted (Fordyce, 1976). Walking and riding a bicycle should therefore be measured in terms of distance, because time spent performing these activities does not provide a measure of how often the component behaviors are performed. Specific exercises, such as deep knee bends, should be quantified in terms of the number of repetitions of that exercise. The exercise or exercises chosen as target behaviors should be those that increase the patient's strength and mobility while doing no structural damage and they should be selected by professionals trained in physical medicine such as physiatrists and physical therapists. To assess exercise tolerance, patients are asked to perform the target exercise ". . . until pain, weakness, or fatigue causes him or her to wish to stop" (Fordyce, 1976, p. 170). Exercise tolerance may be assessed over time as an index of treatment effectiveness.

Mobility

Physical mobility may be measured in many different ways. Three common measures include the straight leg raise, long-sitting to toes, knees to chest (cf. Newman, Seres, Yospe, & Garlington, 1978). In the straight leg raise, patients lay on their backs and lift their legs up as far as possible, keeping the legs straight. The distance between the tips of their fingers and their toes constitutes the measure. Knees to chest is assessed by having patients lay on their back and raise their knees to their chest as far as they can. Mobility is then measured as the degree of hip flexion. As with the mechanical devices, the assessment of physical performance provides an excellent means of gauging treatment outcome, especially for interventions designed specifically to increase the patient's range of motion and flexibility.

COMBINED BEHAVIORAL ASSESSMENT

Although each pain behavior listed in Table 6.1 can be considered distinct and therefore worthy of individual assessment, an overall measure of the construct of pain behavior may be helpful in understanding the degree to which pain influences a variety of related outcome indices.

The only standardized measure that assesses behavior from more than one of the categories presented in Table 6.1 is the University of Alabama (UAB) Pain Behavior Scale (Richards, Nepomuceno, Riles, & Suer, 1982). The UAB scale taps 10 behaviors using 3-point scales. Eight of the rated behaviors are pain communication behaviors: vocal complaints — verbal, vocal complaints — non-verbal, facial grimaces, standing posture, mobility, body language, use of visible supportive equipment, and stationary movement. These eight behaviors are observed using a 5-minute structured observation procedure during which patients are asked to walk, stand, move from a sitting to a standing position, and move from a standing to a sitting position. The two other behaviors rated on the UAB scale are medication use and downtime (from the previous day). The 10 ratings are summed into an overall pain behavior score that may range from 0 to 10.

Two advantages of the UAB scale are its rapid scoring and its demonstrated reliability. Because of the ease of administration, the UAB scale may be employed to gauge pain behavior on a daily basis, thus providing representative observation samples. However, there are two problems with the scale. First, validity data for the scale are lacking: behaviors assessed using the UAB have yet to be compared with alternative measures of the same behaviors. Second, pain communication behaviors are overrepresented in the scale, 8 of the 10 behaviors assessed, suggesting that the UAB should not be considered a comprehensive measure of pain behavior.

The UAB scale is an excellent first step toward the development of a comprehensive measure of pain behavior. Further development of this or similar scales should lead to a more complete understanding of the behavioral aspects of pain and of their relationship to the multiple dimensions of the pain experience.

Chapter 7
The Clinical Pain Interview

The clinical pain interview, while providing a useful method for assessing Context I and II dimensions, is especially useful for selecting and clarifying Context III issues. Based on interview data, Context I information such as diagnosis and medication use and Context II measures such as pain intensity, pain behaviors, and pain cognitions can be placed in their proper developmental and motivational perspectives.

Several discussions of clinical pain interview procedures can be found in the literature (cf. Blanchard & Andrasik, 1985; Catchlove & Ramsay, 1983; Karoly, 1985; Turk & Kerns, 1983). Perhaps the most complete set of ideas are provided by Turk, Meichenbaum, and Genest (1983), who present the clinical pain interview as an integral part of pain treatment. The interview procedure to be presented follows from their suggestions as well as from our own experience with pain patients.

The clinical interview may be divided into five parts: (a) interview questionnaire; (b) interview with the patient and significant other(s); (c) assignment of in vivo assessment tasks; (d) follow-up interview(s), if indicated; and (e) preparation for treatment, if indicated. A brief description of the major issues assessed during each part of the interview is presented in Table 7.1.

INTERVIEW PROCEDURE

Preinterview Questionnaire

The preinterview questionnaire is made up of questions often asked during the course of a regular interview. However, the questions are limited to those that require relatively easy responses. The advantage of a preinterview questionnaire is that much background information can be obtained with relatively little interviewer time.

Figure 7.1 presents a copy of a preinterview questionnaire. Each clinician and interviewer may add or subtract questions depending on the time available to the patient as well as the relative importance of specific questions.

103

Table 7.1   Aspects of the Clinical Pain Interview

I.   *Preinterview Questionnaire Administration*

   A.   Give the patient a preinterview questionnaire that seeks information from several areas of the patient's life (demographic information, pain description data, effects of pain on daily functioning, compensation/litigation status, and pain-coping information).
   B.   Review the questionnaire before the interview begins and note any incomplete responses.

II.   *Interview with the Pain Patient and Significant Other(s)*

   A.   Inquire about questions on the preinterview questionnaires that do not have complete answers.
   B.   Employ a semistructured interview to make sure all important issues are addressed. Important areas to cover include:
      1. Description and history of the pain.
      2. Prior treatments for pain and their effects (as perceived by the patient).
      3. Effects of pain on family relationships.
      4. Special mental health or interpersonal relationship concerns.
   C.   Talk to the significant other(s) who accompany the patient in order to corroborate information obtained from the patient regarding the effects of pain on family relationships and about the manner in which family members are responsible to the patient.

III   *Assignment of In Vivo Assessment Tasks*

   A.   Provide the patient with enough pain diaries (see Chapter 6) to record daily pain levels, positions, medication use, and activities until the next interview. Explain the importance of recording data four times a day rather than once a day. Provide a rationale for the use of the diary (e.g., to understand temporal aspects of pain, to understand how pain is affecting daily life, to serve as a pretreatment measure of quality of life variables, to provide information necessary for the development of a treatment plan, etc.).
   B.   Provide the patient with enough functional assessment diaries (see Chapter 6) to last until the next assessment session (at least two per day). Provide a rationale for the importance of the diary for the understanding and treatment of the patient's pain, and provide detailed and clear instructions in using the diary.
   C.   If possible, provide the patient's major significant other with enough pain diaries to record his or her perception of the patient's pain levels, positions, medication use, and activities. This serves to corroborate patient records and also to increase the accuracy of the patient's self-monitoring. Emphasize the necessity of completing the diaries independently (i.e., without looking at the patient's records or conferring with the patient). Provide detailed instructions and a rationale for using the diary.

IV.   If the patient returns for follow-up assessments and/or treatment sessions, use this opportunity to clarify information obtained in previous assessments.
   A.   Answer questions.
   B.   Review data obtained from the preinterview questionnaire and first interview and be sure you have complete responses to all of the items. Obtain any necessary additional information.
   C.   Review in vivo assessment assignments with the patient and the significant other(s). Reinforce adherence to the assessment tasks. Inquire about any problems the patient had with self-monitoring and discuss how these difficulties may be resolved in the future. Discuss the necessity of continued self-monitoring to provide baseline measures.

D. Review the results of any standardized questionnaires given.
　　1. If the Minnesota Multiphasic Personality Inventory (MMPI) was given (see Chapter 4), note critical items that may require further inquiry.
　　2. Examine any measures of psychopathology given (e.g., scale scores on the MMPI, the Beck Depression Inventory, or the State–Trait Anxiety Inventory, see Chapter 4). If high levels of psychopathology are suggested, inquire about specific symptoms and find out how these may interfere with the patient's life and/or exacerbate pain.

V. *Preparation for Future Treatment*
　　A. Answer questions about your approach to pain treatment.
　　B. Describe your conceptualization/philosophy of pain and its treatment. Indicate how the treatment you provide fits this model and what you expect the outcome of treatment to be (e.g., how will you and the patient know if the treatment is successful).
　　C. Explain what you will do as a treatment provider and what you expect of the patient during treatment. Make clear which of your expectations you consider requisite for a successful outcome (e.g., continued self-monitoring, following through on homework, etc.).
　　D. Set treatment goals. Negotiate goals with both the patient and significant other(s) in areas most in need of change (e.g., social activity, job-related behaviors, and pain-coping efforts). Physical goals such as exercise regimens should be set with appropriate treatment providers (e.g., physical therapist and physician).

Note. Much of the information provided in this table is adapted from Turk, Meichenbaum, & Genest (1983).

Interview With the Patient and Significant Other(s)

The initial contact with the patient can set the tone for the emergent assessment and treatment relationship. From the onset, the assessor should be attempting to form a therapeutic alliance with the patient (Turk, Meichenbaum, & Genest, 1983). This involves listening carefully to patients so as to unearth their questions and concerns about the assessment and treatment process and discussing those concerns openly in order to resolve them.

Along with most other clinicians and researchers (cf. Blanchard & Andrasik, 1985; Catchlove & Ramsay, 1983; Turk, Meichenbaum, & Genest, 1983), we see the development and use of a semistructured interview as the best method for gathering information about a pain patient. The consistent use of an interview protocol means that all patients will be asked specific questions that have been found to be important in problem assessment and in the development of treatment plans.

Interview protocol questions should include those which: (a) the interviewer believes the patient will be unable or unwilling to answer without the assistance of a skilled interviewer (those that patients can respond to on their own should be on the preinterview questionnaire), or (b) will likely require further detailed elaboration or probing.

Demographic information

1. Full name: _____

2. Today's date: _____

3. Your age: _____; Your date of birth: _____

4. Nature of your illness: _____

Present living situation

5. Current marital status (circle one):

   Single   Married   Divorced   Separated   Widowed

6. Who currently lives with you?

Name	*Age*	*Relationship*

7. How is your present living situation different from the way it was before you first experienced pain problems?

   _____

Description of your pain

8. On a scale of 0 to 100, with 0 meaning "no pain" and 100 meaning "pain as bad as it could be", how much pain do you have *on the average*?   _____

9. On the same scale of 0 to 100, how much pain do you have when it is *at its worst*?   _____

10. How much pain do you have when it is *at its least*?   _____

FIGURE 7.2.   Suggested items for a preinterview questionnaire.*

11. How much pain do you have *right now*? _____

12. What seems to make your pain worse (such as: time of day, too much or too little activity, boredom, etc.)? _____

13. What events seem to be associated with decreases in your pain? _____

Effects of pain on daily functioning

14. How many hours *per day* (i.e., in a 24-hour period) do you usually spend out of bed? _____

15. What do you do for a living? _____

16. If you are currently not working:
    A. Are you a full-time homemaker? _____
    B. Are you not working for reasons other than your pain problem? What other reasons?

17.

Question	Before Pain	Now
Hours per week you spend working at a paying job		
Hours per week you spend working at a volunteer job		
Hours per week you spend doing household chores		

18. Are you:
    A. Currently receiving compensation (disability insurance)? _____

    If yes, how much do you receive monthly? $_____

    B. Currently in the process of trying to obtain compensation (disability insurance)? _____

19. Are you involved in any litigation (are you suing anyone) related to your pain (circle one number)?

    1. I have no suit pending.
    2. I am in the process of suing the state or an insurance company to receive compensation benefits for my pain.
    3. I am in the process of suing an individual because he or she is somewhat/totally responsible for my pain problem.

Pain-coping strategies

20. Using the scale below, please indicate how often you use the pain-coping strategy
    listed to control your pain (if you have never heard of or used a particular skill, then
    circle "0" for "never").

Activity	Never	Once a month or less	About once a week	2–4 times week	About once a day	More than once
Biofeedback/ Relaxation	0	1	2	3	4	5
Exercise	0	1	2	3	4	5
Bedrest	0	1	2	3	4	5
Group therapy	0	1	2	3	4	5
Medications	0	1	2	3	4	5
Ignore the pain	0	1	2	3	4	5
TNS unit	0	1	2	3	4	5
Brace	0	1	2	3	4	5
Individual therapy	0	1	2	3	4	5
Heat	0	1	2	3	4	5
Massage/Rubbing	0	1	2	3	4	5

21. Using the scale below, please indicate how effective each pain-coping strategy is
    for you. If you do not use the pain-coping strategy now, indicate how effective *you*
    think the strategy would be for your pain if you were to use it.

Activity	Not at all effective	A little effective	Fairly effective	Mostly effective	Completely effective
Biofeedback/ Relaxation	0	1	2	3	4
Exercise	0	1	2	3	4
Bedrest	0	1	2	3	4
Group therapy	0	1	2	3	4
Medications	0	1	2	3	4
Ignore the pain	0	1	2	3	4
TNS unit	0	1	2	3	4
Brace	0	1	2	3	4
Individual therapy	0	1	2	3	4
Heat	0	1	2	3	4
Massage/Rubbing	0	1	2	3	4

22. If you take medications to control your pain, please indicate below which ones you
    use.

Name of medication	Dose	Average number taken per day

23. What else do you do to control your pain?

_____

24. What do you think should be done about your pain?

_____

Description of the Pain Problem

It is reasonable to begin the interview by focusing on the patient's experience of pain. This may help to alleviate the patient's fear that the assessor believes the pain is not real, or is subordinate to certain psychological matters, such as secondary gain. Of particular importance are the temporal and developmental aspects of pain. We ask how the patient's pain changes over the course of a typical day or week. In addition, it is important to understand the circumstances of pain onset and the duration of suffering per episode.

Because pain can have such a profound influence on a patient's vocational, medical, and social status, we suggest the inclusion of questions in the interview to discern possible impact on each of these areas. We recommend that the assessor discuss the patient's vocational, medical, and social status both before and after the initiation of the pain problem. Furthermore, we ask the question (associated with the diagnostic approach of Alfred Adler): What would your life be like if you did not have to contend with any pain?

---

*On the actual preinterview questionnaire, enough space is provided for the patient to answer the questions.

In addition, we highly recommend that the patient be asked how he or she expects to be functioning in various life areas in the future (in 1 month, 6 months, 1 year, and 5 years). The patient's responses to such questions provide the clinician with three important kinds of information. First, it reveals the patient's current expectations regarding how pain treatment, the patient's own efforts, or both will affect the quality of his or her life. Second, the patient's expectations for the future may also reveal evaluative performance standards. That is, if the patient has become resigned to the prospect of being unemployed for the next 5 years, it may well be difficult to generate much motivation about treatments designed to increase vocational opportunities, even if at some level the patient does wish to get back to work. Third, these questions allow the clinician to discover the rationality of the patient's premises regarding his or her pain problem.

A complete history of past treatments for pain and their effects (as perceived by the patient) provides important data which may help predict future treatment responses and point to the possible use of treatments that have not yet been tried. Have the treatments focused more on psychological or physiological aspects of the problem? If a treatment has been tried, was it continued even when no relief was forthcoming (e.g., repeated operation with no relief) or was it given just a cursory trial?

Effects of Pain on Family Relationships

Because of the potential involvement of the family in the patient's pain problem, we devote a whole section of the interview to addressing familial issues (a Context III issue). We are particularly interested in discovering how the pain problem has improved or, more often, impaired the quality of family relationships. We ask the patient and the family members present to describe how their relationships have changed before and after pain onset in terms of the quantity and quality of time spent together. In terms of spousal relationships, we ask about changes in sexual activities and in feelings about each other. We find it helpful to understand how the patient's role as a parent has changed before and after pain onset in terms of disciplining and nurturing children. Clinical judgments about familial interaction time should be based on knowledge of normative trends as well as idiosyncratic patterns. If a parent with chronic pain reports spending 1 hour with his or her child per day, the assessor should not assume a threat to effective parenting. It has been estimated that parents spend only about 15 minutes per day of quality time with their children. Chronic pain patients may therefore be in a position to improve their familial communication patterns as a result of their household confinement.

We also ask patients and family members how the patient transmits pain information and how the family members respond when they see or hear the patient's message. These questions provide an initial and relatively informal assessment of the patient's pain behaviors in relation to his or her family and also provides the clinician with an initial assessment of the specific reinforcers the patient may be receiving for pain and pain behavior. Such information is helpful when one of the goals of treatment is to assist the patient to alter self-defeating pain behavior, and it may indicate the degree to which family involvement in treatment is necessary. (We find that there are times when it is not necessary to include family members, although we usually attempt to involve the family as much as possible in pain treatment.)

Other Concerns

Only after we have focused on the pain do we initiate a discussion of other concerns. Of particular interest to us has been the assessment of two potential causes of pain exacerbation: emotional turmoil and stressful relationships with others. The link between pain and negative affect is strong. However, because pain patients are sometimes told that their pain is in their head, many are hesitant to admit to emotional difficulties. The appropriate assessment and treatment of these difficulties is an important element in reducing the patient's pain and suffering. Therefore, when inquiring about negative affect, it is a good idea to make clear that emotional concerns are normal. We have found that giving the patient a choice of negative feelings also can encourage the patient to speak openly. The assessor may say:

> Very often patients who have the kind of pain you describe begin to have strong negative feelings about their situation. They often begin to feel a little anxious or hopeless. Which of these feelings do you feel more often? Tell me about how that feels to you? When do you feel the other feeling?

Patients often are experiencing stressful relationships with family members, friends, or co-workers. Unless we specifically ask about these relationships, a potentially important stressor is overlooked, effectively making that aspect of the patient's life unavailable for intervention. We, therefore, always take the time to inquire about relationships, particularly with persons outside of the home.

Follow-up Questions

The last part of the interview consists of questions designed to clarify information already obtained. First we take time to clarify those responses to the preinterview questionnaire which are not complete. We then examine the patient's responses to several specific items of the preinterview questionnaire and expand the information that the patient provided. Specifically we are interested in knowing how aware the patient is of events that increase pain (e.g., does the patient focus only on physical events, or is the patient aware of psychological events that trigger pain episodes?) In addition, we inquire about how the patient uses knowledge of events that trigger pain. Does the patient employ this knowledge to restrict activities or to make it possible to live as fulfilling a life as possible?

Because the patient's compensation and litigation status may influence motivation for treatment, it is important to clearly understand the current legal picture. After reading over the patient's responses on the preinterview questionnaire to the questions that address these issues, we ask the patient to tell us his or her status again during the interview and probe for more details about any litigation or compensation pending.

Finally, we inquire about alcohol use. Rather than ask the patient if he or she drinks alcohol, we ask how much alcohol is consumed. By indicating to the patient that we expect him or her to be regularly using at least some alcohol, we make it a little easier for the patient to admit to alcohol use. It is also important to find out how effective the patient perceives alcohol to be in controlling pain. We have found that many patients, even when they use alcohol to help them forget the pain, state that the alcohol makes them feel more pain in the long run—"I pay for it the next day, believe me!" If there is some indication of alcohol abuse, we arrange for a complete alcohol screening by an individual trained in the assessment and treatment of alcoholism to determine if treatment for alcoholism is indicated before treatment for pain. If the patient does not appear to be abusing alcohol to the point where it is interfering with his or her daily functioning, but may be using alcohol as a pain medication, we may recommend that the appropriate use of alcohol be incorporated in the treatment plan.

Assignment of In Vivo Assessment Tasks

If the assessor has the luxury of seeing the patient more than once, the pain diaries described in chapter 6 may be used to obtain a more direct measure of the events associated with pain episodes and how pain is related to the patient's day-to-day functioning.

In assigning any homework, three things should be kept in mind. First, the patient should not be allowed to take on any homework assignments that he or she has not agreed to complete, at least for the period between sessions. It is important to set the expectation of adherence to homework assignments from the start. Therefore, we will not allow patients to *try* to work on completing diaries. If they do not express a willingness to actually complete the diaries between the time we initially provide the diaries and the next session, we simply state that we will not give the patient any diaries to complete. This approach rarely results in patients not being given diaries, and we have found that it increases adherence to the self-monitoring tasks.

Second, it is important to provide clear instructions for diary keeping, carefully explaining to the patient what is expected. Because these instruments can be complicated, we usually ask the patient to repeat the instructions to make sure they fully understand them.

Finally, we emphasize to the patient the importance of self-monitoring to the understanding and treatment of their particular pain problem. Patients should be given a clear rationale for each step of the task. For example, we tell patients that persons record their behavior more accurately when they record more often, and this is why we expect them to record their activities, position, and medication use four times a day, rather than only at the end of the day.

When possible, we also give the patient's significant other a set of diaries to complete. This serves two functions. First, it provides corroborative data for the variables assessed by the pain diary. Second, it should increase the accuracy of the patient's self-monitoring, because accuracy rates increase when it is known that someone else is observing the same behaviors. When both the patient and a significant other are monitoring the patient's behavior, they should be instructed not to discuss their monitoring results with each other, to insure that independent measures of the patient's behavior are obtained.

It is important to end the interview in a way that will prepare the patient to cooperate even more fully in the interview (whether by the same interviewer or some other interviewer) or in treatment.

One way to end the interview is to request that patients tell you anything about their pain that *they* think is important and about which you have not yet inquired. This offers the patients an opportunity to provide their perspective of their pain in an open-ended format. The interviewer should listen carefully to the patient at this time, because the patient may be more invested in this information that in any other information provided thus far in the interview. Finally, we give patients a chance to ask any questions about the interview or our role in their assessment and treatment. We answer these questions as best we can, sometimes suggesting where they may obtain information about their pain that we are unable or not qualified to provide. Only after we have allowed patients to talk about their pain in an unstructured way and to ask questions of us do we thank them for their time and send them on their way.

Review of In-Session and In Vivo Assessments

If the patient is returning for a follow-up session, then the assessor has the opportunity to review with the patient the data that have been collected so far, as well as to obtain any additional information.

It is wise to begin the follow-up assessment session by asking the patient if he or she has any questions or concerns about the assessment procedure so far. If these questions and concerns are addressed right away, any potential detrimental effects they might have had may be alleviated.

A review of the in vivo assessments is essential. First, the patient and/or significant other should be praised for completing observations as instructed. If the patient was unable to complete the homework assignments as instructed, we attempt to quickly find out what deterred the patient from the self-monitoring task. We do not dwell on nonadherence. With the patient, we make a judgment on his or her ability to follow through on the self-monitoring task before the next session. If together we judge that the patient will complete the self-monitoring as instructed, then we provide additional diaries to be completed. Otherwise, we simply do not use diaries with the patient for a period of time.

Finally, responses to standardized measures of psychopathology are examined and areas of concern are addressed. For example, responses to the Minnesota Multiphasic Personality Inventory (MMPI) (see Chapter 4), if available, may suggest several avenues of inquiry during an interview. Individual items on the MMPI may indicate severe psychological symptoms. Responses to critical items (cf. Lacher & Wrobel, 1979) should be followed up (e.g., some responses may indicate that the patient is considering self-injury and others reveal unusual or bizarre thought processes). In addition, high scores on the clinical scales of the MMPI or other scales (e.g., the Sympton Checklist-90 and the Beck Depression Inventory) (see Chapter 4) should be followed up by further probes concerning the expressed psychopathology and its potential association with the patient's pain problem.

PREPARATION FOR TREATMENT

If the patient will be returning for pain treatment, the end of the interview may be used to prepare the patient for interventions to come.

It is particularly important to provide the patient with your conceptualization of pain, and how the treatment you intend to provide fits this conceptualization. Informing the patient of what to expect allows them to decide whether the treatment fits their needs and prepares them to think of their pain problem as potentially treatable.

Develop a contract with the patient, explicitly writing down what is expected from the treatment provider and from the patient over the course of training, and having both parties sign the contract. Alternatively, the treatment provider may simply state verbally the role he or she will play during the course of treatment and describe what is expected from the patient if treatment is to be successful. Successful treatment should be defined when the philosophy of the treatment is outlined in the form of explicit goals.

The specific treatment goals set depend to a large degree on the treatment(s) offered by the clinician as well on the status and resources of the patient. However, we have found that specification of short-term attainable treatment goals is desirable. It should be emphasized that both the patient and his or her family should be intimately involved in setting the goals, because both have a large investment in and influence on the outcome of treatment. The setting of treatment goals with everyone present helps to promote the therapeutic alliance that is so necessary in the treatment of chronic pain.

CONCLUDING COMMENTS

In this chapter, we have emphasized the importance of the clinical pain interview in obtaining measures from several pain contexts and especially in understanding the patient in terms of Context III dimensions.

Performing an adequate clinical pain interview is not easy. The interview will tax the most skilled clinician, both during the interview, when some patients may not want to discuss issues not directly related to their medical status, and after the interview, when the clinician is expected to make sense of the data collected. In addition, an interview can be time-consuming if complete answers for all of the relevant questions are obtained.

We have found, however, that the information gleaned from a complete interview more than makes up for the time and effort such an interview takes. If the goal of assessment is limited to simply obtaining Context I and II measures for research purposes, as is necessary when pre- and post-treatment measures are needed, then many of the questions recommended in the present chapter become unnecessary. Therefore, it is important for the clinician to carefully consider what will be done with the data collected in deciding (a) whether or not an interview is required, and (b) if so, what questions should be included.

Chapter 8
The Selection and Integration of Pain Measures

The pain assessor who works within a behavioral-science tradition, especially when borrowing models from social and clinical psychology and psychiatry, must be careful not to approximate the stereotype of the tender-minded scientist, of which there are presumably only two types: "those who are frequently wrong but never in doubt, and those who say 'Well it's all very complex', and then hang up the phone" (Shweder & Fiske, 1986, p. 6). Over the years, conceptions of pain have been both oversimplified and paralyzingly intricate, leaving the assessor to negotiate either narrow passageways or broad boulevards in search of a practical perspective. Thus, we encounter many clinicians who administer to their parents nothing but periodic visual analogue scales of intensity and an MMPI, and others who follow the "multiplicity assumption" that it is always best to engage in multiple assessments by multiple assessors at multiple times and places of multiple aspects of pain to achieve a valid and reliable assessment. Ironically, it is just as unworkable to have too much as too little data about a patient, particularly when the contents of the information stockpile turn out to be inconsistent, contradictory, or just plain confusing.

In Chapter 1 we sought to move the field of algesimetry past the categorical approach toward a dynamic, contextual model consistent with the pioneering work of Melzack and Wall (1965), Sternbach (1968), Fordyce (1976), and others. The focus on the immediate, unpleasant sensation of pain with its short-term physical, behavioral, and affective consequences was expanded outward toward the social-vocational world, and inward toward the cognitive representational plane. A major implication of this enlarged framework is its legitimization of diverse, multifaceted assessment strategies including the interview, behavioral observation methods, standardized tests and self-ratings, and biophysical analyses, in addition to biomedical testing (the material of Chapters 2 through to 7). Our goal, however, has not been to give the pain assessor more to do, although it would appear that we have tacitly endorsed a "more is better" philosophy of assessment.

In this final chapter we shall attempt to set the record straight by considering how pain measures might be selected and how varied data sources might be integrated into a coherent picture.

WHAT TO ASSESS, WHY, AND BY WHAT MEANS?

Studies of clinical assessment practices among professionals in various disciplines have shown that preferred measurement strategies and instrumentation often derive from past experience, familiarity with techniques, and a concern for saving time. In other words, clinicians use the methods they have used before and with which they can make relatively rapid decisions with a fairly high degree of confidence. Although we would hardly deny the importance of striving for expert knowledge in any domain, we can suggest that the economy of "prepackaged" assessment is often bought at the expense of diagnostic flexibility. In pain assessment, as in other areas, the avenues explored and the methods used to explore them should be determined by the unique circumstances of the client and the purposes of the assessment.

Based on the conceptual and methodological discussions we have presented thus far, we can point to at least 10 relatively distinct classes of pain information that a clinician may potentially investigate, including data on neurobiological (health) status; pain's impact on functional performance (vocational, avocational, sexual); sensory-perceptual experience; cognitive-evaluational components; affective correlates of pain; on life events and their impact on pain; pain's impact on social and familial functioning; the patient's premorbid competence and adjustment; the patient's potential for medical compliance; and on the patient's potential for self-directed pain management. Obviously, not all of the assessment procedures we have discussed are equally serviceable for obtaining all classes of pain data, nor are all the types of data equally necessary for the management of any given client. Therefore, before we pick our tools, we need to be clear about our assessment goals.

Although we have never seen a statistical tabulation of all the referral questions that accompany pain patients to hospital wards, pain clinics, or private practitioners' offices, we suspect that the most common are: How much pain is the patient really experiencing? Can he or she return to work (school, household duties)? Is the patient a candidate for psychiatric intervention? Is he or she likely to sue me? Can you take this patient off my hands . . . please? Such questions have the virtue of being brief and understandable, although not sufficiently systematic or conceptually compelling to yield equally brief, understandable answers. Conversely, you will recall that in Chapter 1 we made use of the context model (Table 1.1) to suggest that there are fully 49 distinct ways of approaching the question, "What difference does the pain make?" However, between overly general and highly specific interventive and diagnostic questions lies a middle ground of fundamental, boundary-setting clinical objectives to guide our work with pain patients.

Meinhart and McCaffery (1983), borrowing the sociological notion of "pain work" (tasks that occupy health personnel), suggested five general purposes or clinical directions: (a) to diagnose the cause(s) of pain, (b) to control pain expression by the patient, (c) to help the patient endure pain, (d) to help minimize or prevent pain, and (e) to give pain relief. Each of these would involve its own set of specific objectives, the pursuit of which, according to Meinhart and McCaffery, can be managed according to the acronym SOAPIE, which stands for *subjective* and *objective assessment*, followed by the formulation of a *plan* of *intervention*, whose effectiveness is then *evaluated*. Turk and Meichenbaum (1984) suggested another set of five functional tasks of pain work, growing out of their cognitive-behavioral perspective. Their functions include: (a) the collection of baseline information against which to monitor client progress; (b) the gathering of information about the nature of the client's medical condition, previous treatment, illness expectations, and self-perceptions concerning ability to handle pain; (c) the establishment of treatment goals; (d) the initiation of patient education concerning the situational and psychological factors that have impact on the nature and degree of pain; and (e) the clarification of the role of significant others in the maintenance of pain lifestyles, and the determination of their potential as therapeutic change agents.

In sum, it can be said that we assess pain to describe and understand its nature, antecedents, and/or consequences, as well as to plan and evaluate its treatment. The kinds of assessment subgoals we establish, beyond the descriptive and interventive (prescriptive) levels, are a function of our conceptual models. For example, four of the five objectives articulated by Meinhart and McCaffery (1983) have to do with the provision of service. Turk and Meichenbaum's list highlights the importance of placing pain in the context of the patient's life situation and personal resources. Table 8.1 presents a more differentiated list of assessment objectives suggested by the context and control models discussed in Chapter 1.

Obviously, not all of the methods of assessment considered in this book are equally suited to all the potential assessment objectives. Matching one's method to one's clinical question is, however, rarely a serious stumbling block. Limitations on the clinician's time and issues of cost often rule out certain procedures such as in vivo behavioral observation, physiological recording, or diary methods. Furthermore, certain assessment purposes, such as the establishment of a performance baseline for the evaluation of change, tend to indicate certain classes of pain data, such as that concerned with functional performance, pain perception, and affective arousal, as well as particular pain

Table 8.1   Clinical Objectives in the Nonmedical Assessment of Chronic Pain

1.   Identification and preliminary classification of the pain problem (acute vs chronic).
2.   Clarification of medical history and its impact on current expectations, plans, and goals.
3.   Quantification of the disruptiveness versus the benefits of the pain problem in social, marital, and vocational arenas.
4.   Estimation of the patient's premorbid functioning (motoric, social, cognitive, etc.).
5.   Priorizing the foci of the initial intervention(s).
6.   Establishment of a performance baseline from which to evaluate change.
7.   Evaluation of the patient's resources (coping skills, social support systems, etc.).
8.   Clarification of the situational antecedents and cognitive mediators of pain reactivity.
9.   Differentiation of the situational from the sensory antecedents of pain.
10. Selection of intervention strategies matched to patient needs and resources.
11. Forecasting of possible negative side effects of successful treatment.
12. Determination of programmatic treatment alterations.
13. Assessment of posttreatment lifestyle modification.
14. Regulation of the patient's use of pain/nonpain medications.
15. Evaluation of the patient's satisfaction with the pain treatment program(s).
16. Evaluation of familial satisfaction with the pain treatment program(s).
17. Assessment of the patient's self-regulatory motives and skills, particularly in regard to pain control.
18. Assessment of the nature and adjustive impact of the patient's implicit pain theory (schema, scripts, model).

Note.   Adapted from P. Karoly (1985), The assessment of pain: Concepts and issues. In P. Karoly (Ed.), *Measurement Strategies in Health Psychology.* New York: Wiley.

assessment methodologies, such as behavioral observation techniques and subjective pain estimates. Errors in clinical decision-making result more often from a restriction of assessment methods to those that are most familiar or most convenient to use, than from an inability to select an appropriate assessment modality.

The assessor generally tends to acquire a more thorough or complete picture of the pain problem with the use of a variety of distinct assessment modes. However, the use of multimethod assessment carries the potential danger of eliciting data that do not on the surface appear internally consistent or congruent (cf. Nay, 1979). The primary problem with a "more is better" philosophy of measurement is that with the inevitable incongruence in the data comes an all-too-common set of interpretive shortcuts, most of which qualify as examples of diagnostic self-deception. In many clinical assessment contexts, what passes for data integration is better described as an uninspired, dogmatic, and shortsighted search for sameness. "Well, let's see", says the harried clinician, "the MMPI suggests a hypochondriacal pattern, data on health care utilization supports the view of the patient as enacting a 'sick role', yet the patient's activity levels are high and he claims (during interviews) that he wants to 'get back to work and stop thinking so much about his back aches'." How might these findings be treated in decision-making? A number of alternative resolutions are possible, including: counting (two objective indices *for* versus one index *against* the premise that the patient is exaggerating his problems for secondary gain), discounting (You can't trust self-report data!), and second guessing (The interview is more prone to dissimulation than an MMPI, plus everyone knows the interviewer is soft-hearted). Like the mythological Procrustes who sawed off the legs of his guests so as to fit them to his bed, some diagnosticians seem more concerned with establishing a superficial consistency in their data than with synthesizing a better understanding out of seemingly disparate ingredients.

We believe that three related interpretive principles can aid the pain assessor in the process of data integration. These heuristic guidelines include (a) the adaptational and transitional perspective, (b) the naturalistic imperative, and (c) the intentional stance.

The Adaptational/Transitional Perspective

We have found it helpful to remind pain assessors that patients who have undergone prolonged suffering have much with which to cope, have many different maneuvers available to accomplish their goals, and can be at any given time in the midst of an up or down period in the overall process of adjustment. Because it is rare that all potential modalities of adaptation (e.g., the cognitive, the physiological, the affective, and the social) will operate in synchrony, we should not be surprised or dismayed by apparent discrepancies in our findings. The processes of making sense and making do in chronic pain should normally be viewed as changeable and changing.

Having already stressed the importance of gauging a patient's emergent understandings of him- or herself and of his or her current life circumstances, it follows that a useful strategy for clarifying irregularities in a life record might involve juxtaposing three classes of information: (a) typical antecedents functionally linked to typical modes of response, (b) typical antecedents functionally linked to atypical modes of response, and (c) the self-defining nature of each. If *b* is more self-defining than *a* (or equally self-defining), then the patient may be said to be in a transitional state relative to his or her previously "normal" mode of pain adaptation. If the atypical response pattern is deemed beneficial to the patient's life adjustment by both the clinician and the patient, then the transitional state can be termed *potentially growth-enhancing*. Transitions may also be considered as *potentially damaging* and *potentially irrelevant* to long-term adaptation. Whatever their direction, the important point about transitional states is that they may be exceedingly helpful in integrating pain assessment data.

Therefore, the patient whose life circumstances — while they prompt him to rely on the health care system (usual mode of response) — reinforce self-help and relatively unconstrained motor activity (unusual mode of response), may be moving toward greater autonomy and self-sufficiency. The MMPI, which does not reflect what a person can do under the proper motivational conditions and which is not sensitive to change or transition, is not likely to lend confirmation to a positive prognosis, particularly if the MMPI was administered at a time when the patient was psychologically vulnerable. Finally, we can point out that if therapeutic interventions are working, our pain patients will increasingly enter into contact with unfamiliar, affectively-charged, challenging situations, all of which require the generation of new rules of thought or conduct or the revision of old rules. Such circumstances do not tend to call forth a unity of organismic expression, and thus the focal pain dimensions are not likely to be in synchrony.

The Naturalistic Imperative

Throughout this guidebook, we have sought to underscore the importance of specifying precisely what one will assess about pain, why (toward what end), and by what means. The transitional perspective reminds us that the question of when to assess can also be important. Now we can add a fifth dimension — where.

Two common and related assumptions about chronic pain might benefit from careful reexamination: (a) that the pain is portable, and (b) that it is an immediately given experience. These assumptions, which seem so self-evidently true in regard to acute pain, certainly do not accord with the systems-oriented, control-theory model of chronic pain presented in Chapter 1. If these assumptions are effectively challenged, then the *where* of pain assessment becomes a key interpretive consideration. In other words, if the experience and meaning of pain can be tied to distinct settings, goals (desired outcomes as well as unpleasant chores), self-evaluative standards, externally set standards, and the like, then it would make sense to assess pain in places that both evoke these varied schematic contents and contain the cues and contingencies that habitually elicit pain behaviors and cognitions.

When it is impractical for the assessor to be in a client's natural environment (such as the home, school, or workplace), it may yet be possible to recreate in the office or clinic an environment that triggers pain schematic memories and response repertoires. An extended interview, involving open-ended questioning and/or role-play reenactments of critical life events, may therefore serve to augment the generalizability of pain assessments.

Discrepancies in the pain record may partly reflect differences associated with conditions of testing. Therefore, thinking naturalistically (the *naturalistic imperative*) may forestall the interpretive problems that result when ward behavior or spouse reports diverge from personality test or physiological data.

The Intentional Stance

Recall that in Chapter 1 it was asserted that pain could be understood not in isolation but in relation to adaptive concerns, such as goals, social rules, theories, expectations, and the other "meaning elements" within Context III. Furthermore, following Dennett's (1978) reasoning, it was suggested that much could be gained by assuming that the patient, like the clinician, is attempting to make sense of his pain and is guided by intentions vis-à-vis his illness. Such a perspective is especially apt when the assessor confronts contradictions in the pain record.

To illustrate the potential value of the intentional stance, let us examine a common assessment dilemma in clinical work with chronic low back pain patients. As the reader will recall, low back pain syndromes are often diagnosed by exclusion, that is, when the physician can find no medical origin, the conclusion is that the pain is purely *functional*, that is, stress or personality related. Unfortunately, when attempts are made to identify personality correlates or to verify the relationship between pain and stress, the findings are often inconclusive and method-specific.

By dividing the universe discretely into organics, functionals, and normals, some assessors continue to deny the possibility of biopsychosocial interaction along with the view that chronic pain experience can depend, in part, on a higher order, context-dependent interpretive set. Might it not be possible that some patients with low back pain are uniformly physically incapacitated, whereas others are "organic" in different ways, at different times, and for different reasons, implying also that they are normal at different times and for various reasons? Flor, Turk, and Birbaumer (1985) found, for example, that patients with chronic back pain displayed elevated paraspinal electro-myographic levels (abnormal back muscle reactivity) only when the stress they experienced was "personally relevant". Therefore, abnormal back muscle response to stress would certainly qualify as an organic problem (worthy of medical attention), but only when psychologically mediated. Similarly, a back pain patient's response to biofeedback, medication, or psychotherapy of his or her rate of exercise compliance, may fluctuate. These fluctuations may depend upon the stage of coping (transitional perspective); the setting (naturalistic imperative); or the particular way in which the therapeutic regimen affects other important life pursuits, or matches current expectations and interpretive schemes (intentional stance). Therefore, it would be useful for pain assessors to gather data, through questionnaire, interview, diary, or laboratory simulation, dealing with beliefs about illness and pain, plans for the future, causal attributions, preferred control strategies and the relationship of pain to self-perception.

Situating a patient's pain problem within the related frameworks of time, place, and meaning can be of considerable value after the assessor has thoroughly decided on what to measure, why, and by what means. In addition, it has been our experience that such guidebook-based wisdom usually must be tempered by heavy doses of sensitivity, good listening skills, patience, and hard work.

Chapter 9
Afterword

In this guidebook, we have offered a conceptual rationale and a comprehensive review of empirically tested procedures for the clinical assessment of chronic pain in adults. As noted in our preface, we chose to omit detailed discussion of two active areas in pain diagnosis — signal detection methods and broad-based cognitive-behavioral procedures — because these approaches are labor intensive and because their adoption would require a working knowledge of concepts and methodologies which cannot adequately be covered in the space allotted. We shall not apologize further for these sins of omission, but will conclude this volume with a brief critique of the field, and look ahead.

In general terms, clinical pain assessors have too closely emulated the fabled drunkard who, having lost his keys in the dark, chose to search for them under a distant street lamp "because the light was better there". Fascination with pain as a sensory experience and with the intricacies of the human nervous system as the supreme input–output, feedback-control system (whose neurochemical dynamics continue to reveal themselves) will surely lead to new and better techniques for the relief of suffering. However, the abiding emphasis on intensity measurement, often using the McGill Pain Questionnaire as the sole standard against which to validate new assessment procedures, unduly confines the field of chronic pain assessment along a temporal axis — concretizing chronic pain as a short-term experience, rather than allowing it to be viewed as a developmentally emergent process; an experiential axis — focusing on the within-body occurrences of pain or on motoric expression, rather than recognizing the adaptive significance of patient's cognitive representations of their bodily feelings and of their motivated presentational styles of pain display; and along a psychometric axis — searching vainly for a simplistic, quantitative accounting that can adequately capture the multidimensional pain experience and the changing pattern of overt and covert reactions that it engenders.

As a result, several important measurement areas have thus far been understudied or neglected, including the following:

Development of a Structured Pain Interview

It sometimes appears as if clinicians and researchers in algesimetry have forgotten that brief, paper-and-pencil tests and inventories are only meant to serve as provisional substitutes for intensive, theory-directed, and treatment-oriented interviews with patients — interviews built on trust, patience, and a recognition of situational constraints. Despite the good start that has been made (cf. Chapter 7, and Turk, Meichenbaum, & Genest, 1983), there remains a general lack of comparability across studies and clinics owing to the absence of standardization in pain interviewing.

The Study of Pediatric Pain

Conceptual, ethical, and pragmatic constraints have generally limited the study of pain to adult subjects or laboratory animals, making pain in children an understudied area, shrouded in myth and misunderstanding, and often approached inappropriately either as a downward extension of data generated from clinical and research work with developmentally mature, verbal, symbol-manipulating, and relatively autonomous organisms (grown-ups) or as an upward extension from work with rats, dogs, and monkeys who have undergone laboratory pain inductions. As Varni, Jay, Masek, and Thompson (1986) have noted:

> Pain in children represents a complex cognitive-developmental phenomenon, involving a number of biobehavioral components that synergistically interact to produce differential levels of pain perception and verbal and nonverbal manifestations (p. 168).

Yet, despite the recognition from many quarters that pediatric pain is important, complex, and seriously neglected, efforts to assess it in both acute and chronic forms have been narrow in scope and focus (unidimensional), largely atheoretical, and minimally cognizant of developmental factors.

Assessment of Pain Self-Regulation Motives and Competencies

Coping strategies, self-talk, biofeedback, exercise, self-hypnosis, cue-controlled relaxation, and the like can be viewed as delimitable skills, which pain patients have occasionally been taught and that occasionally helps them master felt pain. They do not, however, constitute a conceptually meaningful or operational definition of pain self-regulation. Our brief statement in Chapter 1 of the context model, with an information control/action system approach to chronic pain, sought to highlight the transactional relationship between thoughts, feelings, behavioral enactments, and the social world of shared rules, cues, and contingencies. Essentially, we believe that when individuals psychologically regulate or self-manage their pain, they do so by integrating the information that these varied transacting elements carry. The basic unit of analysis in pain self-regulation, therefore, is neither the intrapsychic intention ("I won't take that drink, no matter how much pain I feel") nor the behavioral skill or cognitive tactic designed to minimize the hurt (distraction, relaxation, self-instruction, and the like): it is the relational cognitive mapping of relevant stimulus information, self-image–related goals, acquired skills, and anticipated outcomes. In broad terms, self-regulation is a process of identity negotiation, fueled by the skilled coordination of internal agendas and social/interpersonal constraints. Clinicians will rarely be successful at training self-control over pain if they concentrate their efforts narrowly on skills acquisition or motivational upgrading, bypassing the values and information-processing competencies that underlie the long-run enactment of the role of "well-adjusted person capable of living with pain". The message for pain assessors, then, is to seek to develop reliable methods for measuring both the contents of the information control/action system (e.g., attentional foci, pain-related memories, goals, and expectancies) and the processing mechanisms associated with pain regulation (e.g., propositional logic, decisional heuristics, attributional styles, symbolization, etc.). Only then can a genuine cognitive behavioral assault on chronic pain be achieved.

A LOOK AHEAD

Although there are gaps in the *what* and *how* of pain assessment, the field nonetheless moves forward. With the advent of multidisciplinary pain programs (evaluations of more than 60 such treatment approaches have been published to date), assessors and intervention agents have been drawn beyond the limits of their specialized training. Increasingly, the effects of pain on families, and the effects of families on patient pain displays, have been taken into account. The politics and economics of pain are also coming under increased scrutiny. It would appear that the time for a multiple context viewpoint is at hand.

We anticipate also that the growing rapprochement between the cognitive and clinical sciences will create an atmosphere wherein the analysis of pain as it is felt or seen will be supplemented with a consideration of pain as it is understood by the patient.

The assessment of representational content generally relies on standardized questionnaires or rating tasks and on structured interviews, the latter often in conjunction with time-limited performance tasks (cf. Karoly, 1985; Merluzzi, Glass, & Genest, 1981; Turk, Meichenbaum, & Genest, 1983). We shall briefly consider how various aspects of a patient's orientation toward his or her pain problem might be indexed by such procedures, keeping in mind that mental contents that must be immediately called on in the performance of a task can be considered more accessible than information that must be retrieved from long-term memory (Ericsson & Simon, 1984).

For example, a study conducted by Genest, Meichenbaum, and Turk (reported in Turk, Meichenbaum, & Genest, 1983) involved asking female subjects, who had immersed their hand in a cold water bath maintained at 2°C, to report on everything they had been feeling and thinking during the immersion period "even if it was brief or random, and even if it seems trivial" (p. 103). Each woman saw a videotape replay of herself during the ice-water task to refresh her memory of the event. Each respondent's verbal output was then recorded and transcribed for later analysis. The procedure, described as a *cognitive reconstruction*, is taken to be an index falling between pure recollection, as when subjects complete an inventory asking them to indicate how they typically react in certain situations, and continuous thought monitoring, in which ratings of thoughts or emotions are given contemporaneously with task performance. Reconstructive methods avoid the problem of memory bias associated with recall tasks and of potential performance interference associated with concurrent verbal reporting.

The key question of course, is: What did Genest and his colleagues learn, in their attempt to assess the content of their subjects' cognitions during a painful procedure? After separating their subjects into two groups, those who tolerated the pain close to the maximum allowable time (300 seconds) and those who kept their hand immersed 100 seconds or less, the authors found that participants

> in the high tolerance group seemed to feel that they could use strategies to affect both the pain and their power to persevere despite the pain, whereas those in the low tolerance group used strategies with less conviction of their usefulness and with less sense of their own ability to influence their situation . . . they (high tolerance subjects) tended to see pain as a problem to be solved rather than as an occasion to engage in negative self-referent ideation of catastrophizing thoughts and images (Turk, Meichenbaum, & Genest, 1983, p. 104).

Keeping in mind that the task used by Genest and his colleagues is analogous to acute rather than chronic pain, the foregoing experiment nonetheless illustrates the possibility that instilling self-confidence and eliminating negativity might prove to be useful therapeutic objectives with chronic pain patients. It further illustrates that "getting inside the heads" of pain patients might be *feasible* as well as clinically productive when done in concert with other assessment procedures.

Based on their extensive experience with cognitive–behavioral pain interventions, Turk, Holzman, and Kerns (1986) found that a common element in successful programs is the provision of a conceptualization or rationale for treatment which patients can understand, accept, and believe. This suggests that a necessary, but probably not a sufficient, goal of cognitive content assessment would be the periodic measurement of patients' models or theories of pain and pain management by means of performance-driven interviews or questionnaires. For example, it has been suggested (Lau & Hartman, 1983; Leventhal, Meyer, & Nerenz, 1980; Leventhal & Nerenz, 1983) that patients can conceptualize illness in accordance with one of three basic schemas: the acute model, in which the illness, or in our case the pain, has a specific cause and is of brief duration; the cyclic model, in which the cause is recurring and the problem persists; or the chronic model, in which there are complex, multiple causes of long duration. Furthermore, within any model, the problem may be articulated along five dimensions: identity, consequence, time line, cause, and cure. Among the most common clinical observations of chronic pain patients is their tendency to retain an acute pain model within which the expectation of a cure for a definable, physical, and not a psychological or interpersonal, disorder persists in the face of much counterevidence. In accordance with the control theory model, it has been hypothesized (Karoly, 1985) that the attempt to eliminate or suppress the sensation of pain, consistent with an acute model, is incompatible with effective day-to-day management of pain. Readers are referred to Leventhal and Nerenz (1985) for a more complete discussion of methods for the assessment of patients' so-called commonsense models of illness.

We further anticipate an increased reliance on the part of pain assessors upon procedures which can preserve or index the sequences, transactions, and/or functional relationships between pain-relevant thoughts, feelings, behaviors, and setting conditions. The use of diaries for in vivo naturalistic assessment should see continued development. Laboratory-based performance tasks (simulations) can also address the processes of pain perception and control, rather than being limited to capturing only end points. Most laboratory studies have been limited, however, by their rather unilateral focus on measures of pain endurance, failing to take into account events associated with attention, representation, evaluation, goal-setting, and the self-directed control over pain and its affective correlates.

The CoPAP Paradigm

In our laboratories at Arizona State University, we have been developing a simulation paradigm that we feel addresses each of the two aforementioned main weaknesses of laboratory analogue approaches to the study of self-directed pain control. Predicated on several compatible conceptual models, the procedure seeks to examine the manner by which individuals manage not only painful sensations but correlated emotional states, and (most importantly from a Context III standpoint) also examines ongoing performance levels on a task in which they have some personal investment. On the negative side, the paradigm, which we refer to as CoPAP, for *control* of *pain*, *affect*, and *performance*, uses cold pressor (ice water) pain induction, which stimulates acute rather than chronic suffering, and performance motivation is experimentally rather than naturally primed. However, we believe the CoPAP paradigm comes closer than previous arrangements to possessing a minimal degree of ecological validity. It was designed to meet each of the 10 criteria listed in Table 9.1.

The criteria reflect the multiple context and information/action control approach to pain outlined in Chapter 1 of this volume, a cognitive social learning model of self-control (Kanfer, 1986; Kanfer & Hagerman, 1981; Karoly & Kanfer, 1982), and motivation-based theories of action regulation (cf. Frese & Sabini, 1985; Hacker, 1985; Heckhausen & Kuhl, 1985; von Cranach, Machler, & Steiner, 1985). Essentially, these conceptualizations emphasize the importance of examining pain relationally, that is, in relation to various self- and other-set standards, in relation to tangible goal pursuits, in relation to information-processing differences, in relation to attentional focus, self-appraisal, and attribution, in relation to various task-relevant cognitions, and over time. The multiple context approach, particularly Context III, advises us to uncover the adaptive significance of pain for work-related and cognitive performance. The control theory model emphasizes the temporal processing of pain signals and their cognitive representations. Models of self-control tell us to be aware of multiple sources of feedback about performance and of the self-corrective maneuvers (both cognitive and behavioral, and covert and publicly observable) that can keep the actor on course toward a goal, even when staying on course literally hurts.

The criteria proposed therefore involve the performance of an ego-involving task in competition with another person; the examination of moods; the inclusion of stable (trait-like) and fluctuating (state) variables; the setting and

Table 9.1   Criteria for a Comprehensive Laboratory Simulation of Self-Directed Pain/Affect/Performance Control

1.	An achievement-oriented setting should be established (e.g., performance matters to the participant(s); a competitive set exists)
2.	Physical pain capable of interfering with task performance and/or intentions should be induced
3.	Ongoing performance appraisal should be subject to multiple (alternative) standards of self-motivation
4.	Some self-evaluative standards should be capable of generating negative affective states (e.g., depression, anxiety, anger, shame)
5.	The affective states engendered in the experiment should be periodically assessed and their relationship to performance determined
6.	Relevant stylistic differences in schematic information processing should be assessed before performance
7.	The content of subjects' goals and actions (including level of task achievement, persistence, change in pain tolerance, change in affective arousal) should be assessed over time (trials)
8.	Both temporally variable and static (structural) indices of pain/affect/performance control should be included
9.	Both covert (cognitive, emotive, imaginal) and overt (behavioral) indices of pain and affect control should be included
10.	Some aspects of performance feedback should be under experimental control

resetting of performance goals (intentions); and the examination of changes (over trials) in patterned relations among variables both "under the skin" and in the immediate environment — a reflection of a landscape that is more like the real world, we believe, than the picture printed in previous laboratory studies of pain and its control.

Perhaps the only criterion in need of further discussion is number 3, that when the subject is appraising his performance, it should not be in reference to a single evaluative standard. For the most part, laboratory investigators of pain control have given the subject nothing else to do but to try to tolerate pain for increasingly long periods of time. Although certainly not an unimportant goal, the focus on endurance, or its correlates, misses the very critical point that pain sufferers not only need to tolerate pain but also continue to engage in other life tasks — some trivial and some important, waxing and waning in their consciousness — and they are rarely free to put everything else on hold. Multiple performance objectives suggest multiple standards. Indeed, even a single performance objective (e.g., "Keep my hand immersed in the ice-water bath as long as I can") can be evaluated from several distinct perspectives (e.g., Beat my best time; Beat my worst time; Beat the best time obtained by a peer; Beat some ideal time by an imagined other; "Don't tolerate the ice-water any longer than I have been commanded to by an authority", etc.) (cf. Higgins, Strauman, & Klein, 1986, for a more complete discussion of the mutiplicity of evaluative standards that individuals are capable of enacting). Therefore, the priming and assessment of different standards will be an important ingredient in helping to bring the laboratory closer to real life.

References

Adams, J., Brechner, V. L., & Brechner, T. (1979). The reliability of some techniques utilized in quantifying the intensity of clinical pain. *Pharmacology and Therapeutics, 4*, 629–632.

Adriaensen, H., Gybels, J., Handwerker, H. O., & Van Hees, J. (1984). Suppression of C-fibre discharges upon repeated heat stimulation may explain characteristics of concomitant pain sensations. *Brain Research, 302*, 203–211..

Agnew, D. C., & Merskey, H. (1976). Words of chronic pain. *Pain, 2*, 73–81.

Ahles, T. A., Ruckdeschel, J. C., & Blanchard, E. B. (1984). Cancer-related pain. II. Assessment with visual analogue scales. *Journal of Psychosomatic Research, 28*, 121–124.

Akil, H., Richardson, D. E., Hughes, J., & Barchas, J. D. (1978). Enkephalin-like material elevated in ventricular cerebrospinal fluid of pain patients after analgetic focal stimulation. *Science, 201*, 463–465.

Akil, H., Watson, S. J., Young, E., Lewis, M. E., Khachaturian, H., & Walker, J. M. (1984). Endogenous opiods: Biology and function. *Annual Review of Neuroscience, 7*, 223–255.

Almay, B. G. L., Johansson, F., VonKnorring, L., Terenus, L., & Wahlström, A. (1978). Endorphins in chronic pain. I. Differences in CSF endorphin levels between organic and psychogenic syndromes. *Pain, 5*, 153–162.

Andrasik, F., Blanchard, E. B., Ahles, T., Pallmeyer, T., Barron, K. D. (1981). Assessing the reactive as well as the sensory component of headache pain. *Headache, 21*, 218–221.

Andrasik, F., Blanchard, E. B., Arena, J. G., Saunders, N. L., & Barron, K. D. (1982) Psychophysiology of recurrent headache: Methodological issues and new empirical findings. *Behavior Therapy, 13*, 407–429.

Andrasik, F., & Holroyd, K. A. (1980). Physiologic and self-report comparisons between tension headache sufferers and nonheadache controls.. *Journal of Behavioral Assessment, 2*, 135–141.

Appenzeller, O. (1969). Vasomotor function in migraine. *Headache, 9*, 147–155.

Appenzeller, O., Davison, K., & Marshall, J. (1963). Reflex vasomotor abnormalities in the hands of migrainous subjects. *Journal of Neurology and Neurosurgical Psychiatry, 26*, 447–450.

Armentrout, D. P., Moore, J. E., Parker, J. C., Hewett, J. E., & Feltz, C. (1982). Pain-patient MMPI subgroups: The psychological dimensions of pain. *Journal of Behavioral Medicine, 5*, 201–211.

Bailey, J. O., Jr., McCall, W. D. Jr., & Ash, M. M., Jr. (1977). Electromyographic silent periods and jaw motion parameters: Quantitative measures of temporomandibular joint dysfunction. *Journal of Dental Research, 56*, 249–253.

Bakal, D. A. (1975). Headache: A biopsychological perspective. *Psychological Bulletin, 82*, 369–382.

Bakal, D. A., & Kaganov, J. A. (1977) Muscle contraction and migraine headache: Psychophysiologic comparison. *Headache, 17*, 208–215.

Beck, A. T., Rush, A. J. Shaw, B. F., & Emery, G. (1979). *Cognitive therapy of depression.* New York: Guilford.

Beecher, H. K. (1959). *Measurement of subjective responses: Quantitative effects of drugs.* New York: Oxford University Press.

Belkin, S. (1985) Back pain. In G. M. Aronoff (Ed.), *Evaluation and treatment of chronic pain.* Baltimore: Urban & Schwarzenberg.

Bergner, M., Bobbitt, R. A., Carter, W. B., & Gilson, B. S. (1981). The sickness impact profile: Development and final revision of a health status measure. *Health Care, 19*, 787-805.

Bessette, R., Bishop, B., & Mohl, W. (1971). Duration of masseteric silent period in patients with TMJ syndrome. *Journal of Applied Physiology, 30*, 864-869.

Bessette, R. W., Mohl, N. D., & Di Cosimo, C. J., II. (1974). Comparison of results of electromyographic and radiographic examinations in patients with myofascial pain-dysfunction syndrome. *Journal of the American Dental Association, 89*, 1358-1364.

Blanchard, E. B., & Andrasik, F. (1985). *Management of chronic headaches: A psychological approach*. Elmsford, N.Y.: Pergamon.

Block, A. R., Kremer, E., & Gaylor, M. (1980a). Behavioral treatment of chronic pain: Variables affecting treatment efficacy. *Pain, 8*, 367-375.

Block, A. R., Kremer, E. F., & Gaylor, M. (1980b). Behavioral treatment of chronic pain: The spouse as a discriminative cue for pain behavior. *Pain, 9*, 243-252.

Blumer, D., & Heilbronn, M. (1981). The pain-prone disorder: A clinical and psychological profile. *Psychosomatics, 22*, 395-402.

Bonica, J. J. (1981). Preface. In K. Y. Lorenz (Ed.), *New approaches to the treatment of chronic pain*. Washington, DC: National Institute on Drug Abuse.

Bradley, L. A., & Van der Heide, L. H. (1984). Pain-related correlates of MMPI profile subgroups among back pain patients. *Health Psychology, 3*, 157-174.

Brena, S. F. (1983). The medical diagnostic process. In S. F. Brena & S. L. Chapman (Eds.), *Management of patients with chronic pain*. New York: SP Medical & Scientific Books.

Brodman, K., Erdmann, A. J., Lorge, I., & Wolff, H. G. (1949). The Cornell Medical Index: An adjunct to medical interview. *Journal of the American Medical Association, 140*, 530-534.

Brown, G. K., & Nicassio, P. M. (1985, November). *Development of a questionnaire for assessing active and helpless coping strategies in chronic pain patients*. Paper presented at the 19th annual convention of the Association for the Advancement of Behavior Therapy, Houston, TX.

Budzynski, T. H., Stoyva, J. M., Adler, C. S., & Mullaney, D. J. (1973). EMG biofeedback and tension headache: A controlled outcome study. *Psychosomatic Medicine, 35*, 484-496.

Burckhardt, C. S. (1984). The use of the McGill Pain Questionnaire in assessing arthritis pain. *Pain, 19*, 305-314.

Byrne, M., Troy, A., Bradley, L. A., Marchisello, P. J., Geisinger, K. F., Van der Heide, L. H., & Prieto, E. J. (1982). Cross-validation of the factor structure of the McGill Pain Questionnaire. *Pain, 13*, 193-201.

Cairns, D., Thomas, L., Mooney, V., & Pace, J. B. (1976). A comprehensive treatment approach to chronic low back pain. *Pain, 2*, 301-308.

Catchlove, R. F. H., & Ramsay, R. A. (1983). A protocol for the medico-psychosocial evaluation of patients with chronic pain. *Canadian Anaesthetists Society Journal, 30*, 531-535.

Chapman, C. R., Casey, K. L., Dubner, R., Foley, K. M., Gracely, R. H., & Reading, A. E. (1985). Pain measurement: An overview. *Pain, 22*, 1-31.

Chapman, C. R., Chen, A. C. N., & Harkins, S. W. (1979). Brain evoked potentials as correlates of laboratory pain: A review and perspective. In J. J. Bonica, J. C. Liebeskind, & D. G. Albe-Fessard (Eds.), *Advances in pain research and therapy: Vol. 3*. New York: Raven.

Chapman, C. R., & Wyckoff, M. (1981). The problem of pain: A psychobiological perspective. In S. N. Haynes & L. Gannon (Eds.), *Psychosomatic disorders: A psychophysical approach to etiology and treatment*. New York: Praeger.

Charter, R. A., & Nehemkis, A. M. (1983). The language of pain intensity and complexity: New methods of scoring the McGill Pain Questionnaire. *Perceptual and Motor Skills, 56*, 519-537.

Chen, A. C. N., Chapman, C. R., Harkins, S. W. (1979). Brain evoked potentials are functional correlates of induced pain in man. *Pain, 6*, 365-374.

Chen, A. C. N., Treede, R. D., & Bromm, B. (1984). Modulation of pain evoked cerebral potential by concurrent subacute pain. In B. Bromm (Ed.), *Pain measurement in man: Neurophysiological correlates of pain* (pp. 301-310). Amsterdam: Elsevier.

Chesney, M. A. & Shelton, J. L. (1976). A comparison of muscle relaxation and electromyogram biofeedback treatments for muscle contraction headache. *Journal of Behavior Therapy and Experimental Psychiatry, 7*, 221-225.

Chudler, E. H., & Dong, W. K. (1983). The assessment of pain by cerebral evoked potentials. *Pain, 16*, 221-244.

Cinciripini, P. M., & Floreen, A. (1982). An evaluation of a behavioral program for chronic pain. *Journal of Behavioral Medicine, 5*, 375-389.

Cinciripini, P. M., & Floreen, A. (1983). An assessment of chronic pain behavior in a structured interview. *Journal of Psychosomatic Research, 27*, 117-123.

Cleeland, C. S., Shacham, S., Dahl, J. L., & Orrison, W. (1984). CSF beta-endorphin and the severity of pain. *Neurology, 34*, 378-380.

Cohen, R. A., Williamson, D. A., Monguilott, J. E., Hutchinson, P. C., Gottlieb, J., & Waters, W. F. (1983). Psychophysiological response patterns in vascular and muscle-contraction headaches. *Journal of Behavioral Medicine, 6*, 93-107.

Collins, F. L., & Thompson, J. K. (1979). Reliability and standardization in the assessment of self-reported headache pain. *Journal of Behavioral Assessment, 1*, 73-86.

Cram, J. R. & Steger, J. C. (1983). EMG scanning in the diagnosis of chronic pain. *Biofeedback and Self-Regulation, 8*, 229-241.

Crisson, J., Keefe, F. J., Wilkins, R. H., Cook, W. A., & Muhlbaier, L. H. (1986). Self report of depressive symptoms in low back pain patients. *Journal of Clinical Psychology, 42*, 425-430.

Crockett, O. J., Prkachin, K. M., & Craig, K. D. (1977). Factors of the language of pain in patient and volunteer groups. *Pain, 4*, 175-182.

Crue, B. L. (Ed.). (1979). *Chronic pain.* New York: Spectrum.

Crue, B. L. (1983). The neurophysiology and taxonomy of pain. In S. F. Brena & S. L. Chapman (Eds.), *Management of patients with chronic pain.* New York: SP Medical & Scientific Books.

Crue, B. L. (1985). Forward. In G. M. Aronoff, (Ed.), *Evaluation and treatment of chronic pain.* Baltimore: Urban & Schwarzenberg.

Dennett, D. C. (1978). *Brainstorms: Philosophical essays on mind and psychology.* Cambridge, Massachusetts: MIT Press.

Derogatis, L. R. (1977). *The SCL-90-R:* Administration scoring and procedures manual I. Baltimore: Clinical Psychometric Research.

Diener, E. (1984). Subjective well-being. *Psychological Bulletin, 95*, 542-575.

Dolce, J. J., & Raczynski, J. M. (1985). Neuromuscular activity and electromyography in painful backs: Psychological and biomechanical models in assessment and treatment. *Psychological Bulletin, 97*, 502-520.

Donchin, E., McCarthy, G., Kutas, M., & Ritter, W. (1983). Event-related brain potentials in the study of consciousness. In R. J. Davidson, G. E. Schwartz, & D. Shapiro (Eds.), *Consciousness and self-regulation: Advances in research and theory: Vol. 3.* New York: Plenum.

Downey, J. A., & Frewin, D. B. (1972). Vascular responses in the hands of patients suffering from migraine. *Journal of Neurology, Neurosurgery, and Psychiatry, 35*, 258-263.

Downie, W. W., Leatham, P. A., Rhind, V. M., Wright, V., Branco, J. A., & Anderson, J. A. (1978). Studies with pain rating scales. *Annals of the Rheumatic Diseases, 37*, 378-381.

Dubuisson, D., & Melzack, R. (1976). Classification of clinical pain descriptions by multiple group discriminant analysis. *Experimental Neurology, 51*, 480-487.

Duckro, P. N., Margolis, R. B., & Tait, R. C. (1985). Psychological assessment in chronic pain. *Journal of Clinical Psychology, 41*, 499-504.

Elliott, K., Frewin, D. B., & Downey, J. A. (1974). Reflex vasomotor responses in the hands of patients suffering from migraine. *Headache, 13*, 188-196.

Elton, D., Burrows, G. D., & Stanley, G. V. (1979). Clinical measurement of pain. *Medical Journal of Australia, 1*, 109-111.

Elton, D., Stanley, G., & Burrows, G. (1983). *Psychological control of pain.* Sydney: Grune & Stratton.

Engel, G. L. (1959). Psychogenic pain and the pain-prone patient. *American Journal of Medicine, 26*, 899-918.

Engelbart, H. J., & Vrancken, M. A. E. (1984). Chronic pain from the perspective of health: A view based on systems theory. *Social Science and Medicine, 19*, 1383-1392.

Epstein, L. H., & Abel, G. G. (1977). An analysis of biofeedback training effects for tension headache patients. *Behavior Therapy, 8*, 37-47.

Epstein, L. H., Abel, G. G., Collins, F., Parker, L., & Cinciripini, P. M. (1978). The relationship between frontalis muscle activity and self-reports of headache pain. *Behavior Research and Therapy, 16*, 153-160.

Ericsson, K. A., & Simon, H. A. (1984). *Protocol analysis: Verbal reports as data.* Cambridge, Massachusetts: MIT Press.

Feuerstein, M., Bortolussi, L., Houle, M., & Labbé, E. (1983). Stress, temporal artery activity, and pain in migraine headache: A prospective analysis. *Headache, 23,* 296–304.

Flor, H., & Turk, D. C. (1984). Etiological theories and treatments for chronic back pain. I: Somatic models and interventions. *Pain, 19,* 105–121.

Flor, H., Turk, D. C., & Birbaumer, N. (1985). Assessment of stress-related psychophysiological reactions in chronic back pain patients. *Journal of Consulting and Clinical Psychology, 53,* 354–364.

Folkard, S., Glynn, C. J., & Lloyd, J. W. (1976). Diurnal variation and individual differences in the perception of intractable pain. *Journal of Psychosomatic Research, 20,* 289–301.

Follick, M. J., Ahern, D. K., & Aberger, E. W. (1985). Development of an audiovisual taxonomy of pain behavior: Reliability and discriminant validity. *Health Psychology, 4,* 555–568.

Follick, M. J., Ahern, D. K., & Laser-Wolston, N. (1984). Evaluation of a daily activity diary for chronic pain patients. *Pain, 19,* 373–382.

Follick, M. J., Ahern, D. K., Laser-Wolston, N., Adams, A. E., & Molloy, A. J. (1985). Chronic pain: Electromechanical recording device for measuring patients' activity patterns. *Archives of Physical Medicine and Rehabilitation, 66,* 75–79.

Follick, M. J., Smith, T. W., & Ahern, D. K. (1985). The Sickness Impact Profile: A global measure of disability in chronic low back pain. *Pain, 21,* 67–76.

Fordyce, W. (1976). *Behavioral methods for chronic pain and illness.* St. Louis: C. V. Mosby.

Fordyce, W. E. (1979). *Use of the MMPI in the assessment of chronic pain.* New Jersey: Hoffman La Roche.

Fordyce, W. E., Fowler, R. S., Jr., Lehmann, J. F., DeLateur, B. J., Sand, P. L., & Trieschmann, R. B. (1973). Operant conditioning in the treatment of chronic pain. *Archives of Physical Medicine and Rehabilitation, 54,* 399–408.

Fox, E. J., & Melzack, R. (1976). Trancutaneous electrical stimulation and acupuncture: Comparison of treatment for low-back pain. *Pain, 2,* 141–148.

Frank, A. J. M., Moll, J. M. H., & Hort, J. F. (1982). A comparison of three ways for measuring pain. *Rheumatology and Rehabilitation, 21,* 211–217.

French, E. B., Lassers, B. W., & Desai, M. G. (1967). Reflex vasomotor responses in the hands of migrainous subjects. *Journal of Neurology and Neurosurgical Psychiatry, 30,* 276–278.

Frese, M., & Sabini, J. (Eds.). (1985). *Goal-directed behavior: The concept of action in psychology.* Hillsdale, NJ: Lawrence Erlbaum.

Fries, J. F., Spitz, P., Kraines, R. G., & Holman, H. R. (1980). Measurement of patient outcome in arthritis. *Arthritis and Rheumatism, 23,* 137–145.

Fries, J. F., Spitz, P. W., & Young, D. Y. (1982). The dimensions of health outcomes: The Health Assessment Questionnaire, Disability and Pain scales. *Journal of Rheumatology, 9,* 789–793.

Gannon, L. R., Haynes, S. N., Safranek, R., & Hamilton, J. (1981). A psychophysiological investigation of muscle-contraction and migraine headache. *Journal of Psychosomatic Research, 25,* 271–280.

Garron, D. C., & Leavitt, F. (1979). Demographic and affective covariates of pain. *Psychosomatic Medicine, 41,* 525–534.

Garron, D. C., & Leavitt, F. (1983). Chronic low back pain and depression. *Journal of Clinical Psychology, 39,* 487–493.

Gatchel, R. J., Deckel, A. W., Weinberg, N., & Smith, J. E. (1985). The utility of the Millon Behavioral Health Inventory in the study of chronic headaches. *Headache, 25,* 49–54.

Genazzani, A. R., Nappi, G., Facchinetti, F., Micieli, G., Petraglia, F., Bono, G., Monittola, C., & Savoldi, F. (1984). Progressive impairment of CSF ß-EP levels in migraine sufferers. *Pain, 18,* 127–133.

Gergen, K. J. (1985). Social constructionist inquiry: Context and implications. In K. J. Gergen & K. E. Davis (Eds.), *The social construction of the person.* New York: Springer-Verlag.

Gildenberg, P. L., & DeVaul, R. A. (1985). *The chronic pain patient: Evaluation and management.* Basel: S. Karger.

Götestem, K. G., & Linton, S. J. (1985). Pain. In M. Hersen & A. S. Bellack (Eds.), *Handbook of clinical behavior therapy with adults.* New York: Plenum.

Gotlib, I. H. (1984). Depression and general psychopathology in university students. *Journal of Abnormal Psychology, 93,* 19–30.

Gottlieb, H., Strite, L. C., Koller, R., Madorsky, A., Hockersmith, V., Kleeman, M., & Wagner, J. (1977). Comprehensive rehabilitation of patients having chronic low back pain. *Archives of Physical Medicine and Rehabilitation, 58*, 101–108.

Gracely, R. H., McGrath, P., & Dubner, R. (1978a). Ratio Scales of sensory and affective verbal pain descriptors. *Pain, 5*, 5–18.

Gracely, R. H., McGrath, P., & Dubner, R. (1978b). Validity and sensitivity of ratio scales of sensory and affective verbal pain descriptors: Manipulation of affect by diazepam. *Pain, 5*, 19–29.

Graham, C., Bond, S. S., Gerkovich, M. M., & Cook, M. R. (1980). Use of the McGill Pain Questionnaire in the assessment of cancer pain: Replicability and consistency. *Pain, 8*, 377–387.

Gross, A. R. (1986). The effect of coping strategies on the relief of pain following surgical intervention for lower back pain. *Psychosomatic Medicine, 48*, 229–241.

Gross, R. T., & Collins, F. L., Jr. (1981). On the relationship between anxiety and pain: A methodological confounding. *Clinical Psychology Review, 1*, 375–386.

Hacker, W. (1985). On some fundamentals of action regulation. In G. P. Ginsburg, M. Brenner, & M. von Cranach (Eds.), *Discovery strategies in the psychology of action*. London: Academic.

Hall, W. (1981). On "ratio scales of sensory and affective verbal pain descriptors." *Pain, 4*, 101–107.

Hallin, R. G. (1984). Human pain mechanisms studied with percutaneous microneurography. In B. Bromm (Ed.), *Pain measurement in man. Neurophysiological correlates of pain*. Amsterdam: Elsevier.

Hawkins, R. P., & Dobes, R. W. (1977). Behavioral definitions in applied behavior analysis: Explicit or implicit? In B. C. Etzel, J. M. LeBlanc, & D. M. Baer (Eds.), *New developments in behavioral research: Theory, method, and application*. Hillsdale, NJ: Erlbaum.

Haynes, S. N., Griffin, P., Mooney, D., & Parise, M. (1975). Electromyographic biofeedback and relaxation instructions in the treatment of muscle contraction headaches. *Behavior Therapy, 6*, 672–678.

Heckhaussen, H., & Kuhl, J. (1985). From wishes to action: The dead ends and short cuts on the long way to action. In M. Frese & J. Sabini (Eds.), *Goal-directed behavior*. Hillsdale, NJ: Erlbaum.

Hendler, N., Uematsu, S., Long, D. (1982). Thermographic validation of physical complaints in 'psychogenic pain' patients. *Psychosomatics, 23*, 283–287.

Hendler, N., Viernstein, M., Gucer, P., & Long, D. (1979). A preoperative screening test for chronic back pain patients. *Psychosomatics, 20*, 801–808.

Higgins, E. T., Strauman, T., & Klein, R. (1986). Standards and the process of self evaluation: Multiple affects from multiple stages. In R. M. Sorrentino & E. T. Higgins (Eds.), *Handbook of motivation and cognition*. New York: Guilford.

Hockaday, J. M., Macmillan, A. L., & Whitty, C. W. M. (1967). Vasomotor-reflex response in idiopathic and hormone-dependent migraine. *Lancet, 1*, 1023–1026.

Hoon, P. W., Feurstein, M., & Papciak, A. S. (1985). Evaluation of the chronic low back pain patient: Conceptual and clinical considerations. *Clinical Psychology Review, 5*, 377–401.

Hosobuchi, Y., Rossier, J., Bloom, F. E., Guillemin, R. (1979). Stimulation of human periaqueductal gray for pain relief increases immunoreactive beta-endorphin in ventricular fluid. *Science, 203*, 279–281.

Hoyt, W. H., Hunt, H. H., Jr., DePauw, M. A., Bard, D., Shaffer, F., Passias, J. N., Robbins, D. H., Jr., Runyon, D. G., Semrad, S. E., Symonds, J. T., & Watt, K. C. (1981). Electromyographic assessment of chronic low-back pain syndrome. *Journal of the American Osteopathic Association, 80*, 728–730.

Hunter, M. (1983). The headache scale: A new approach to the assessment of headache pain based on pain descriptions. *Pain, 16*, 361–373.

Jacob, R. G., Turner, S. M., Szekely, B. C., & Eidelman, B. H. (1983). Predicting outcome of relaxation therapy in headaches: The role of "depression". *Behavior Therapy, 14*, 457–465.

Jeffrey, D. B. (1974). Self-control: Methodological issues and research trends. In M. J. Mahoney & C. E. Thorsen (Eds.), *Self-control: Power to the person*. Monterey, CA: Wadsworth.

Jensen, M. P., Karoly, P., & Braver, S. (1986). The measurement of clinical pain intensity: A comparison of six methods. *Pain, 27*, 117–126.

Joyce, C. R. B., Zutshi, D. W., Hrubes, V., & Mason, R. M. (1975). Comparison of fixed interval and visual analogue scales for rating chronic pain. *European Journal of Clinical Pharmacology, 8*, 415–420.

Kallman, W. M., & Feuerstein, M. (1977). Psychophysiological procedures. In A. R. Ciminero, K. S. Calhoun, & H. E. Adams (Eds.), *Handbook of behavioral assessment*. New York: John Wiley.

Kanfer, F. H. (1986, April). *Self regulation and behavior*. Paper presented at the Ringberg Symposium on "Volition and Action," Schloss Ringberg, F. R. Germany.

Kanfer, F. H., & Hagerman, S. (1981). The role of self-regulation. In L. Rehm (Ed.), *Behavior therapy for depression: Present status and future directions*. New York: Academic.

Kaplan, R. M., Metzger, G., & Jablecki, C. (1983). Brief cognitive and relaxation training increases tolerance for a painful clinical electromyographic examination. *Psychosomatic Medicine, 45*, 155–162.

Karoly, P. (1985). The assessment of pain: Concepts and issues. In P. Karoly (Ed.), *Measurement strategies in health psychology* New York: John Wiley.

Karoly, P., & Kanfer, F. H. (Eds.). (1982). *Self-management and behavior change*. New York: Pergamon.

Keefe, F. J., & Block, A. R. (1982). Development of an observation method for assessing pain behavior in chronic low back pain patients. *Behavior Therapy, 13*, 363–375.

Keefe, F. J., & Brown, C. J. (1982). Behavioral treatment of chronic pain syndromes. In P. A. Boudewyns & F. J. Keefe (Eds.), *Behavioral medicine in general medical practice*. Menlo Park, CA: Addison-Wesley.

Keefe, F. J., Crisson, J. E., Maltbie, A., Bradley, L., & Gil, K. M. (in press). Illness behavior as a predictor of pain and overt behavior patterns in chronic low back pain patients. *Journal of Psychosomatic Research*.

Keefe, F. J., & Hill, R. W. (1985). An objective approach to quantifying pain behavior and gait patterns in low back pain patients. *Pain, 21*, 153–161.

Keefe, F. J., Wilkins, R. H., & Cook, W. A. (1984). Direct observation of pain behavior in low back pain patients during physical examination. *Pain, 20*, 59–68.

Keefe, F. J., Wilkins, R. H., Cook, W. A., Jr., Crisson, J. E., & Muhlbaier, L. H. (in press). Depression, pain, and pain behavior. *Journal of Consulting and Clinical Psychology*.

Kelly, D. D. (1981). Somatic sensory systems. IV. Central representations of pain and analgesia. In E. R. Kandel & J. H. Schwartz (Eds.), *Principles of neural science*. New York: Elsevier/North Holland.

Kerns, R. D., Turk, D. C., & Rudy, T. E. (1985). The West Haven-Yale Multidimensional Pain Inventory (WHYMPI). *Pain, 23*, 345–356.

Kiser, R. S., Gatchel, R. J., Bhatia, K., Khatami, M., Huang, X., & Altshuler, K. Z. (1983). Acupuncture relief of chronic pain syndrome correlates with increased plasma met-enkephalin concentrations. *Lancet, 2*, 1394–1396.

Kremer, E., & Atkinson, J. H. (1981). Pain measurement: Construct validity of the affective dimension of the McGill Pain Questionnaire with chronic benign pain patients. *Pain, 11*, 93–100.

Kremer, E., Atkinson, J. H., & Ignelzi, R. J. (1981). Measurement of pain: Patient preference does not confound pain measurement. *Pain, 10*, 241–248.

Kremer, E. F., Atkinson, J. H., & Kremer, A. M. (1983). The language of pain: Affective descriptors of pain are a better predictor of psychological disturbance than pattern of sensory and affective descriptors. *Pain, 16*, 185–192.

Kremer, E. F., Sieber, W., & Atkinson, J. H. (1985). Spousal perpetuation of chronic pain behavior. *International Journal of Family Therapy, 7*, 258–270.

Lachar, D. (1974). *The MMPI: Clinical assessment and automated interpretation*. Los Angeles: Western Psychological Services.

Lachar, D., & Wrobel, T. A. (1979). Validating clinician's hunches: Construction of a new MMPI critical item set. *Journal of Consulting and Clinical Psychology, 47*, 277–284.

La Freniere, J. G. (1979). *The low back patient*. New York: Masson.

Lau, R. R., & Hartman, K. A. (1983). Common sense representation of common illnesses. *Health Psychology, 2*, 167–185.

Leavitt, F. (1983). Detecting psychological disturbance using verbal pain measurement: The Back Pain Classification Scale. In R. Melzack (Ed.), *Pain measurement and assessment*. New York: Raven.

Leavitt, F., & Garron, D. C. (1979a). Psychological disturbance and pain report differences in both organic and non-organic low back pain patients. *Pain, 7,* 187–195.

Leavitt, F., & Garron, D. C. (1979b). Validity of a back pain classification scale among patients with low back pain not associated with demonstrable organic disease. *Journal of Psychosomatic Research, 23,* 301–306.

Leavitt, F., & Garron, D. C. (1980). Validity of a back pain classification scale for detecting psychological disturbance as measured by the MMPI. *Journal of Clinical Psychology, 36,* 186–189.

Leavitt, F., Garron, D. C., Whisler, W. W., & Sheinkop, M. B. (1978). Affective and sensory dimensions of back pain. *Pain, 4,* 273–281.

Leavitt, F., Garron, D. C., Whisler, W. W. & D'Angelo, C. M. (1980). A comparison of patients treated by chymopapin and laminectomy for low back pain using a multidimensional pain scale. *Clinical Orthopaedics and Related Research, 146,* 136–143.

LeRoy, P. L., & Bruner, W. M. (1982). Effects of electrical stimulation on the thermographic pattern in the human patient with chronic pain syndrome. *Progress in Clinical and Biologic Research, 107,* 389–395.

LeRoy, P. L., Bruner, W. M., Christian, C. R., Filasky, R., & LeRoy, S. (1985). Thermography as a diagnostic aid in the management of chronic pain. In G. M. Aronoff (Ed.), *Evaluation and treatment of chronic pain.* Baltimore: Urban & Schwarzenberg.

Leventhal, H., & Everhart, D. (1979). Emotion, pain, and physical illness. In C. E. Izard (Ed.), *Emotions in personality and psychopathology.* New York: Plenum.

Leventhal, H., Meyer, D., & Nerenz, D. R. (1980). The common sense representation of illness danger. In S. Rachman (Ed.), *Contributions to medical Psychology: Vol. 2.* New York: Pergamon.

Leventhal, H., & Nerenz, D. R. (1983). A model for stress research with some implications for the control of stress disorders. In D. Meichenbaum & M. Jaremko (Eds.), *Stress reduction and prevention.* New York: Plenum.

Leventhal, H., & Nerenz, D. R. (1985). The assessment of illness cognition. In P. Karoly (Ed.), *Measurement strategies in health psychology.* New York: John Wiley.

Lewis, J. W., Nelson, L. R., Terman, G. W., Shavit, Y., & Liebeskind, J. C. (1986). Intrinsic control mechanisms of pain perception. In R. J. Davidson, G. E. Schwartz, & D. Shapiro (Eds.), *Consciousness and self-regulation: Advances in research and theory: Vol. 4.* New York: Plenum.

Lindblom, V., & Tegner, R. (1979). Are the endorphins active in clinical pain states? Narcotic antagonism in chronic pain patients. *Pain, 7,* 65–68.

Linton, S. J., Melin, L., & Götestam, K. G. (1984). Behavioral analysis of chronic pain and its management. In M. Hersen, R. M. Eisler, & P. M. Miller (Eds.), *Progress in behavior modification: Vol. 18.* New York: Academic Press.

Mahoney, M. J., & Thoresen, C. E. (1974). *Self-control: Power to the person.* Monterey, CA: Brooks/Cole.

Main, C. J., & Waddell, G. (1985). The communication of pain and distress in chronic orthopaedic conditions. In E. Karas (Ed.), *Current issues in clinical psychology: Vol. 2.* New York: Plenum Press.

Mann, S. G., Kimber, G., Diggins, J. B., Jenkins, R. Vandenburg, M. J., & Currie, W. J. C. (1984). Methods of assessing pain in clinical trials. *Clinical Science, 66,* 78.

Marbach, J. J., & Lund, P. (1981). Depression, anhedonia and anxiety in temporomandibular joint and other facial pain syndromes. *Pain, 11,* 73–84.

Margolis, R. B., Tait, R. C., & Krause, S. J. (1986). A rating system for use with patient pain drawings. *Pain, 24,* 57–65.

Martin, J. H. (1981). Somatic sensory systems. II. Anatomical substrates for somatic sensation. In E. R. Kandel & J. H. Schwartz (Eds.), *Principles of neural science.* New York: Elsevier/North Holland.

Martin, P. R., & Mathews, A. M. (1978). Tension headaches: Psychophysiological investigation and treatment. *Journal of Psychosomatic Research, 22,* 389–399.

McCall, W. D., Jr., Uthman, A. A., & Mohl, N. D. (1978). TMJ symptom severity and EMG silent periods. *Journal of Dental Research, 57,* 709–714.

McCreary, C., Turner, J., & Dawson, E. (1979). The MMPI as a predictor of response to conservative treatment for low back pain. *Journal of Clinical Psychology, 35,* 278–284.

McCreary, C., Turner, J., & Dawson, E. (1981). Principal dimensions of the pain experience and psychological disturbance in chronic low back pain patients. *Pain, 11,* 85–92.

McNair, D. M., Lorr, M., & Droppleman, L. F. (1971). *Manual for the profile of mood states.* San Diego: Educational and Industrial Testing Service.

Meinhart, N. T., & McCaffery, M. (1983). *Pain: A nursing approach to assessment and analysis.* Norwalk, CT: Appleton-Century-Crofts.

Melzack, R. (1975). The McGill Pain Questionnaire: Major properties and scoring methods. *Pain, 1,* 277-299.

Melzack, R. (1983). The McGill Pain Questionnaire. In R. Melzack (Ed.), *Pain measurement and assessment.* New York: Raven.

Melzack, R., & Casey, K. L. (1968). Sensory motivational, and central control determinants of pain: A new conceptual model. In D. Kenshalo (Ed.), *The skin senses.* Springfield, IL: Charles C Thomas.

Melzack, R., & Perry, C. (1975). Self-regulation of pain: The use of alpha-feedback and hypnotic training for the control of chronic pain. *Experimental Neurology, 46,* 452-469.

Melzack, R., & Torgerson, W. S. (1971). On the language of pain. *Anesthesiology, 34,* 50-59.

Melzack, R., & Wall, P. (1965). Pain mechanisms: A new theory. *Science, 50,* 971-979.

Melzack, R., & Wall, P. D. (1983). *The challenge of pain.* New York: Basic Books.

Merluzzi, T. V., Glass, C. R., & Genest, M. (Eds.). (1981). *Cognitive assessment.* New York: Guilford.

Merskey, H. (1978). Diagnosis of the patient with chronic pain. *Journal of Human Stress, 4,* 3-7.

Millon, T., Green, C. J., & Meagher, R. B., Jr. (1979). The MBHI: A new inventory for the psychodiagnostician in medical settings. *Professional Psychology, 10,* 529-539.

Moore, P. A., Duncan, G. H., Scott, D. S., Gregg, J. M., & Ghia, J. N. (1979). The submaximal effort tourniquet test: Its use in evaluating experimental and chronic pain. *Pain, 6,* 375-382.

Murphy, J. K., Sperr, E. V., & Sperr, S. J. (1986). Chronic pain: An investigation of assessment instruments. *Journal of Psychosomatic Research, 30,* 289-296.

Nachemson, A. L. (1975). Towards a better understanding of low back pain: A review of the mechanics of the lumbar disc. *Rheumatology and Rehabilitation, 14,* 129-143.

Nachemson, A. L. (1976). The lumbar spine, an orthopedic challenge. *Spine, 1,* 59-71.

Nay, W. R. (1979). *Multimethod clinical assessment.* New York: Gardner Press.

Nelson, R. O. (1977). Methodological issues in assessment via self-monitoring. In J. D. Cone & R. P. Hawkins (Eds.), *Behavioral assessment: New directions in clinical psychology.* New York: Brunner/Mazel.

Newman, R. I., Seres, J. L., Yospe, L. P., & Garlington, B. (1978). Multidisciplinary treatment of chronic pain: Long-term follow-up of low-back pain patients. *Pain, 4,* 283-292.

Nigl, A. J. (1984). *Biofeedback and behavioral strategies in pain treatment.* New York: SP Medical & Scientific Books.

Nystrom, B., & Hagbarth, K. E. (1981). Microelectrode recordings from transected nerves in amputees with phantom limb pain. *Neuroscience Letters, 27,* 211-216.

Oakeshott, M. (1933). *Experience and its modes.* Cambridge: Cambridge University Press.

Oakley, D. A. (1985). Animal awareness, consciousness and self-image. In D. A. Oakley (Ed.), *Brain and mind.* London: Methuen.

Oakley, D. A., & Eames, L. C. (1985). The plurality of consciousness. In D. A. Oakley (Ed.), *Brain and mind.* London: Methuen.

Ohnhaus, E. E., & Adler, R. (1975). Methodological problems in the measurement of pain: A comparison between the verbal rating scale and the visual analogue scale. *Pain, 1,* 379-384.

Peck, R. E. (1967). A precise technique for the measurement of pain. *Headache, 6,* 189-194.

Pilowsky, I. (1967). Dimensions of hypochondriasis. *British Journal of Psychiatry, 113,* 89-93.

Pilowsky, I., Spence, N., Cobb, J., & Katsikitis, M. (1984). The Illness Behavior Questionnaire as an aid to clinical assessment. *General Hospital Psychiatry, 6,* 123-130.

Pinsky, J. (1978). Chronic, intractable, benign pain: A syndrome and its treatment with intensive short-term group psychotherapy. *Journal of Human Stress, 4,* 17-21.

Pinsky, J., & Crue, B. L. (1984). Intensive group psychotherapy. In P. D. Wall & R. Melzack (Eds.), *Textbook of pain.* Edinburgh: Churchill Livingston.

Prieto, E. J., Hopson, L., Bradley, L. A., Byrne, M., Geisinger, K. F., Midax, D., & Marchisello, P. J. (1980). The language of low back pain: Factor structure of the McGill Pain Questionnaire. *Pain, 8,* 11-19.

Ransford, A. O., Cairns, D., & Mooney, V. (1976). The pain drawing as an aid to the psychologic evaluation of patients with low-back pain. *Spine, 1,* 127-134.

Rathus, S. A. (1973). A 30-item schedule for assessing assertive behavior. *Behavior Therapy, 4*, 398–406.

Reading, A. E. (1979). The internal structure of the McGill Pain Questionnaire in dysmenorrhoea patients. *Pain, 7*, 353–358.

Reading, A. E., & Newton, J. R. (1978). A card sort method of pain assessment. *Journal of Psychosomatic Research, 22*, 503–512.

Reich, J., Rosenblatt, R. M., & Tupin, J. (1983). DSM III: A new nomenclature for classifying patients with chronic pain. *Pain, 16*, 201–206.

Richards, J. S., Nepomuceno, C., Riles, M., & Suer, Z. (1982). Assessing pain behaivor: The UAB Pain Behavior Scale. *Pain, 14*, 393–398.

Rosenstiel, A. K., & Keefe, F. J. (1983). The use of coping strategies in chronic low back pain patients: Relationship to patient characteristics and current adjustment. *Pain, 17*, 33–44.

Ross, D. M., & Ross, S. A. (1984). Childhood pain: The school-aged child's viewpoint. *Pain, 20*, 179–191.

Rowat, K. M. (1985). Assessing the "Chronic pain family." *International Journal of Family Therapy, 7*, 284–296.

Roy, R. (1985). The international perspective on pain behavior in marriage. *International Journal of Family Therapy, 7*, 271–283.

Rybstein-Blinchik, E. (1979). Effects of different cognitive strategies on chronic pain experience. *Journal of Behavioral Medicine, 2*, 93–101.

Sanders, S. (1979). Behavioral assessment and treatment of clinical pain: Appraisal of current status. In M. Hersen, R. Eisler, & P. M. Miller (Eds.), *Progress in behavior modification: Vol. 8.* New York: Academic.

Sanders, S. H. (1980). Toward a practical instrument system for the automatic measurement of "up-time" in chronic pain patients. *Pain, 9*, 103–109.

Savitz, D. (1985). Medical evaluation of the chronic pain patient. In G. M. Aronoff (Ed.), *Evaluation and treatment of chronic pain.* Baltimore: Urban & Schwarzenberg.

Scarry, E. (1985). *The body in pain.* New York: Oxford University Press.

Schwartz, D. P., & DeGood, D. E. (1984). Global appropriateness of pain drawings: Blind ratings predict patterns of psychological distress and litigation status. *Pain, 19*, 383–388.

Seymour, R. A. (1982). The use of pain scales in assessing the efficacy of analgesics in post-operative dental pain. *European Journal of Clinical Pharmacology, 23*, 441–444.

Shacham, S., Reinhardt, L. C., Raubertas, R. F., & Cleeland, C. S. (1983). Emotional states and pain: Intraindividual and interindividual measures of association. *Journal of Behavioral Medicine, 6*, 405–419.

Shweder, R. A., & Fiske, D. W. (1986). Introduction: Uneasy social science. In D. W. Fiske & R. A. Shweder (Eds.), *Metatheory in social science: Pluralisms and subjectivities.* Chicago: University of Chicago Press.

Sicuteri, F., Anselmi, B., Curradi, D., Michelacci, S., & Sassi, A. (1978). Morphine-like factors in CSF of headache patients. *Advances in Biochemical Psychopharmacology, 18*, 363–366.

Sjölund, B., Terenius, L., & Eriksson, M. (1977). Increased electro-acupuncture. *Acta Physiologica Scandinavica, 100*, 382–384.

Slade, P. (1985). Theories of chronic pain phenomena. In E. Karas (Ed.), *Current issues in clinical psychology: Vol. 2.* New York: Plenum.

Smukler, N. M. (1985). Pain perception. *Bulletin on the Rheumatic Diseases, 35*, 1–8.

Spielberger, C. D. (1983). *Manual for the State-Trait Anxiety Inventory (Form Y).* Palo Alto, CA: Consulting Psychologists Press.

Stein, N., Fruchter, H. J., & Trief, P. (1983). Experiences of depression and illness behavior in patients with intractable chronic pain. *Journal of Clinical Psychology, 39*, 31–33.

Stenn, P. G., Mothersill, K. J., & Brooke, R. I. (1979). Biofeedback and a cognitive behavioral approach to treatment of myofascial pain dysfunction syndrome. *Behavior Therapy, 10*, 29–36.

Sternbach, R. A. (1968). *Pain: A psychophysiological analysis.* New York: Academic.

Sternbach, R. A. (1974). *Pain patients: Traits and treatment.* New York: Academic.

Sternbach, R. A. (1983). The tourniquet pain test. In R. Melzack (Ed.), *Pain measurement and assessment.* New York: Raven.

Sternbach, R. A., Deems, L. M., Timmermans, G., & Huey, L. Y. (1977). On the sensitivity of the tourniquet pain test. *Pain, 3*, 105–110.

Sternbach, R. A., Wolf, S. R., Murphy, R. W., & Akeson, W. H. (1973). Aspects of chronic low back pain. *Psychosomatics, 14*, 52–56.

Sweet, J. J., Breuer, S. R., Hazlewood, L. A., Toye, R., & Pawl, R. P. (1985). The Millon Behavioral Health Inventory: Concurrent and predictive validity in a pain treatment center. *Journal of Behavioral Medicine, 8*, 215–226.

Terenius, L. (1984). Approaches to neuropeptide and, in particular, endorphin measurement. *Advances in Biochemical Psychopharmacology, 39*, 35–43.

Terenius, L., & Wahlström, A. (1975). Morphine-like ligand for opiate receptors in human CSF. *Life Sciences, 16*, 1759–1764.

Thomas, L. J., Tiber, N., & Schireson, S. (1973). The effects of anxiety and frustration on muscular tension related to the temporomandibular joint syndrome. *Oral Surgery, 36*, 763–768.

Toomey, T. C., Gover, V. F., & Jones, B. N. (1983). Spatial distribution of pain: A descriptive characteristic of chronic pain. *Pain, 17*, 289–300.

Toomey, T. C., Gover, V. F., & Jones, B. N. (1984). Site of pain: Relationship to measures of pain description, behavior and personality. *Pain, 19*, 389–397.

Trief, P. M., & Yuan, H. A. (1983). The use of the MMPI in a chronic back rehabilitation program. *Journal of Clinical Psychology, 39*, 47–52.

Turk, D. C., Holzman, A. D., & Kerns, R. D. (1986). Chronic pain. In K. A. Holroyd & T. L. Creer (Eds.) *Self-management of chronic disease.* Orlando, FL: Academic Press.

Turk, D. C., & Kerns, R. D. (1983). Conceptual issues in the assessment of clinical pain. *International Journal of Psychiatry in Medicine, 13*, 57–68.

Turk, D. C., & Meichenbaum, D. (1984). A cognitive behavioral approach to pain management. In P. D. Wall & R. Melzack (Eds.), *Textbook of pain.* Edinburgh: Churchill Livingstone.

Turk, D. C., Meichenbaum, D., & Genest, M. (1983). *Pain and behavioral medicine.* New York: Guilford.

Turk, D. C., Rudy, T. E., & Flor, H. (1985). Why a family perspective for pain? *International Journal of Family Therapy, 7*, 223–234.

Turk, D. C., Rudy, T. E., & Salovey, P. (1985). The McGill Pain Questionnaire reconsidered: Confirming the factor structure and examining appropriate uses. *Pain, 21*, 385–397.

Turner, J. A. (1982). Comparison of group progressive-relaxation training and cognitive-behavioral group therapy for chronic low back pain. *Journal of Consulting and Clinical Psychology, 50*, 757–765.

Turner, J. A., & Romano, J. M. (1984). Self-report screening measures for depression in chronic pain patients. *Journal of Clinical Psychology, 40*, 909–913.

Tursky, B., Jamner, L. D., & Friedman, R. (1982). The pain perception profile: A psychophysical approach to the assessment of pain report. *Behavior Therapy, 13*, 376–394.

Urban, B. J., Keefe, F. J., & France, R. D. (1984). A study of psychophysical scaling in chronic pain patients. *Pain, 20*, 157–168.

Vallbo, A. B., Hagbarth, K. E., Torebjork, H. E., & Wallin, B. G. (1979). Somatosensory, proprioceptive, and sympathetic activity in human peripheral nerves. *Physiological Reviews, 59*, 919–957.

Varni, J. W., Jay, S. M., Masek, B. J., & Thompson, K. L. (1986). Cognitive-behavioral assessment and management of pediatric pain. In A. D. Holzman & D. C. Turk (Eds.), *Pain management: A handbook of psychological treatment approaches.* New York: Pergamon.

Von Baeyer, C. L., Bergstrom, K. J., Brodwin, M. G., & Brodwin, S. K. (1983). Invalid use of pain drawings in psychological screening of back pain patients. *Pain, 16*, 103–107.

Von Cranach, M., Machler, E., & Steiner, V. (1985). The organisation of goal-directed action: A research report. In G. P. Ginsburg, M. Brenner, & M. Von Cranach (Eds.), *Discovery strategies in the psychology of action.* London: Academic Press.

Wallenstein, S. L., Heidrich, G., III, Kaiko, R., & Houde, R. W. (1980). Clinical evaluation of mild analgesics: The measurement of clinical pain. *British Journal of Clinical Pharmacology, 10*, 3195–3275.

Wallin, G., Torebjork, E., & Hallin, R. (1976). Preliminary observations on the pathophysiology of hyperalgesia in the causalgic pain syndrome. In Y. Zotterman (Ed.), *Sensory function of the skin in primates with special reference to man.* Oxford: Pergamon.

Waring, E. M., Weisz, G. M., & Bailey, S. I. (1976). Predictive factors in the treatment of low back pain by surgical intervention. In J. J. Bonica & D. Albe-Fessard (Eds.), *Advances in pain research and therapy: Vol. 1.* New York: Raven.

Watkins, L. R., & Mayer, D. J. (1982). Organization of endogenous opiate and nonopiate pain control systems. *Science, 216*, 1185–1192.

Weimer, W. B. (1977). A conceptual framework for cognitive psychology: Motor theories of the mind. In R. Shaw & J. Bransford (Eds.), *Perceiving, acting, and knowing: Toward an ecological psychology.* New York: John Wiley.

Weisenberg, M. (1977). Pain and pain control. *Psychological Bulletin, 84*, 1008–1044.

Wildman, B. G., & Erickson, M. T. (1977). Methodological problems in behavioral observation. In J. D. Cone & R. P. Hawkins (Eds.), *Behavioral assessment: New directions in clinical psychology.* New York: Brunner/Mazel.

Wolf, S. L., & Basmajian, J. V. (1978). Assessment of paraspinal electromyographic activity in normal subjects and in chronic back pain patients using a muscle biofeedback device. In E. Asmussen & K. Jorgenson (Eds.), *Biomechanics. VI. Proceedings of the Sixth International Congress of Biomechanics.* Baltimore: University Park Press.

Wolf, S. L., Basmajian, J. V., Russe, C. T. C., & Kutner, M. (1979). Normative data on low back mobility and activity levels: Implications for neuromuscular reeducation. *American Journal of Physical Medicine, 58*, 217–229.

Wolf, S. L., Nacht, M., & Kelly, J. L. (1982). EMG feedback training during dynamic movement for low back pain patients. *Behavior Therapy, 13*, 395–406.

Woodforde, J. M., & Merskey, H. (1972). Some relationships between subjective measures of pain. *Journal of Psychosomatic Research, 16*, 173–178.

Yemm, R. (1969). Temporomandibular dysfunction and masseter muscle response to experimental stress. *British Dental Journal, 127*, 508–510.

Zonderman, A. B., Heft, M. W., & Costa, P. T., Jr. (1985). Does the Illness Behavior Questionnaire measure abnormal illness behavior? *Health Psychology, 4*, 425–436.

Zung, W. W. K. (1965). A self-rating depression scale. *Archives of General Psychiatry, 12*, 63–70.

Author Index

Subject Index

About the Authors

Paul Karoly received his doctorate in clinical psychology from the University of Rochester. Before moving to Arizona State University as Professor and Director of the Clinical Training Program, he served on the psychology faculty of the University of Cincinnati. Dr. Karoly has been an Associate Editor for *Behavior Therapy* and a member of the editorial boards of the *Journal of Personality and Social Psychology, Behavioral Assessment*, and the *Journal of Consulting and Clinical Psychology*. He is currently Associate Editor of *Behavioral Assessment*. He has edited or co-edited nine other volumes, including: *Measurement Strategies in Health Psychology* (1985), *Self-Management and Behavior Change* (1982; with F. H. Kanfer), and *Improving the Long-term Effects of Psychotherapy* (1980; with J. J. Steffen). Dr. Karoly has been extensively involved in research on the mechanisms of functional and dysfunctional self-regulation, children's adaptation to chronic illness, personality and psychopathology, as well as the conceptualization, assessment, and modification of pain.

Mark P. Jensen received his bachelor's degree from Macalester College and is currently completing his doctoral work in clinical psychology at Arizona State University, with a specialization in Health Psychology. He has published several research papers and reviews in the area of health psychology and pain assessment.

Psychology Practitioner Guidebooks

Editors
Arnold P. Goldstein, Syracuse University
Leonard Krasner, Stanford University & SUNY at Stony Brook
Sol L. Garfield, Washington University

Walter B. Pryzwansky & Robert N. Wendt—PSYCHOLOGY AS A PROFESSION: Foundations of Practice

Cynthia D. Belar, William W. Deardorff & Karen E. Kelly—THE PRACTICE OF CLINICAL HEALTH PSYCHOLOGY

Paul Karoly & Mark P. Jensen—MULTIMETHOD ASSESSMENT OF CHRONIC PAIN

William L. Golden, E. Thomas Dowd & Fred Friedberg—HYPNOTHERAPY: A Modern Approach

Patricia Lacks—BEHAVIORAL TREATMENT FOR PERSISTENT INSOMNIA

Arnold P. Goldstein & Harold Keller—AGGRESSIVE BEHAVIOR: Assessment and Intervention

C. Eugene Walker, Barbara L. Bonner & Keith L. Kaufman—THE PHYSICALLY AND SEXUALLY ABUSED CHILD: Evaluation and Treatment

Robert E. Becker, Richard G. Heimberg & Alan S. Bellack—SOCIAL SKILLS TRAINING TREATMENT FOR DEPRESSION